Advance Praise for
Barefoot to Benefactor

"Lenny Peters' faith shines through on every page of his book. It's a faith that can buoy us through the obstacles that keep us from manifesting our life's work, just as it has done for Lenny."

> — **Anthony Atala, M.D.,** Professor and Director of the Wake Forest Institute for Regenerative Medicine, and Chair of the Department of Urology at Wake Forest School of Medicine in North Carolina

"It's so refreshing to read the life story of a man who learns, aspires, and finds creative ways to do good in the world. His faith in God and in others has led to great accomplishments, yet he remains rooted in his humility and generous desire to give. Dr. Peters' memoir encourages our faith and resilience. That is his gift to us."

> — **David Mounts,** Chairman/CEO, Inmar Intelligence

"I dare anyone to read Lenny Peters' life story and not come away with a renewed sense that anything is possible when we believe. A true original, Lenny will inspire you to be your best self."

> — **Roy E. Carroll II,** Owner and CEO, The Carroll Companies

"A wonderful book! Lenny Peters has led a remarkable life that can motivate us all to stay connected to our faith and our communities."

> — **Derek L. Ellington,** Managing Director, Business Banking, Atlantic-South Region Executive, Bank of America

"Lenny's winning memoir recounts how one man, for all of his triumphs, has never forgotten his roots. His story makes anything seem possible, and this uplifting book will inspire you to make the world a better place."

> — **Dave Horne,** Government Relations Lawyer Partner, Smith Anderson Law

"I have often wondered how Dr. Lenny Peters acquired his business acumen, his healing abilities, and his compassion for others—and through this generous memoir, now I know. With his trademark self-deprecation and large-hearted spirit, Dr. Peters relates a life full of blessings that he never takes for granted."

— **Rick Callicutt,** Chairman, Carolinas and Virginia Pinnacle Financial Partners

"Lenny Peters paints a vivid portrait of his childhood in India and how his faith in God moved him to turn obstacles into opportunities, to better himself and those around them. This memoir is a stirring testament to how building yourself can allow you to offer more to others."

— **Paul Mengert,** CEO, Association Management Group

"Lenny's story of coming to America, achieving success, and giving back couldn't be timelier. For anyone looking to unite their Christian values with their professional lives, this book proves it can be done while staying true to oneself."

— **Senator Don Vaughan**, Adjunct Professor of Law, Wake Forest University

Barefoot
to
Benefactor

*My Life Story
of Faith and Courage*

LENNY PETERS, M.D.

Post Hill Press
New York • Nashville
posthillpress.com

Published in the United States of America
1 2 3 4 5 6 7 8 9 10

To my children, Shirin, Elise, Anthony, and Nicole.

Contents

PART V: THROUGH THE POWER OF FORGIVENESS

ACKNOWLEDGMENTS

Self-quarantining at home during the COVID-19 pandemic has had its benefits, allowing me the opportunity to write this book.

A special thanks to my business partner and daughter, Elise Peters Carey, for her commitment to taking my legacy and my spirit to the next generation and beyond.

I would also like to thank J.R. and Matt, my sons-in-law, and Ashley, my daughter-in-law, for their special contributions to our family.

I am grateful and humbled to have been allowed the honor of welcoming into the world, and into our family, my grandchildren, Cosimo, Adeline, Soma, Charlotte, Isabel, Edward, and James.

This book is also dedicated to the many angels without wings who have touched my life and left a positive mark in some way. At every turn, throughout my life and across four continents, these kind souls have unselfishly, with compassion and sometimes with tough love, helped steer me toward greater opportunities and have guided me along this journey toward my destiny.

PRELUDE

I stood still, not moving a fraction of an inch. Inside, I was trembling. I couldn't believe this was happening. Again. Tiny pins pricked ever so slightly with every breath. Still, I knew the result would be stunning. The designer, Luis Machicao, had pinned his exquisite suits on movie stars, world leaders, even royalty. And now he had come to me, hadn't even demanded I fit the suit at his studio as was his custom. Instead, he stood in my bedroom, measuring and pinning, draping and tucking, so that I could wear his original design when I went, once again, to the White House.

Unlike the other times, when I'd been invited to join large events, this time I had been invited for a private meeting with the president, where I would meet the heads of state, the vice president, and their families. Of course, I'd had the honor of meeting such illustrious figures before, but not in such an intimate setting. The suit, this time, had to be perfect. It had to surpass any suit I'd ever worn to meet presidents in the past.

The occasion was Christmas, so the fabric we had selected for the formal jacket was a deep garnet red, with the most subtle brocade woven into its silk threads. The trim, a simple, classic black, matched the stylish black slacks. An elegant but festive suit coat, one that spoke of both wealth and confidence, the confidence to wear red before the most powerful man in the world.

"Nice suit," the president would later say, taking the fabric between his fingers. "I'd like a jacket like this. Where can I get one made?"

"Mr. President," I answered with pride, "I shall have a suit like this made especially for you."

He smiled, pleased. He pulled me aside and introduced me to other prominent figures. We spoke about India, my home country. Earlier, at the reception of two hundred people, all dignitaries, senators, and wealthy patrons, I was struck to see I was the only Indian among them. Not like prior events at the White House. This time, I alone represented my home country.

Later in the evening, speaking with the chief of staff, I asked, "Where is the Indian ambassador? I seem to be the only Indian here."

"Oh, he wasn't invited," he answered, shrugging his shoulders. "You're more important."

Whether flattery or truth, it didn't matter. I swelled with pride, marveling at how far I had come in the six decades since my birth. Could I ever have imagined I would be in private company with the president of the United States?

And yet from the start I somehow knew that that had been exactly the destiny before me. It was the universe that led the way.

PART I

MY DESTINY BEGINS

"Success is not final, failure is not fatal. It is the courage to continue that counts."

Sir Winston Churchill

❧ CHAPTER 1 ❧

A Garden of Eden on the Arabian Sea

I like to win. More precisely, I like to meet any challenge that comes my way. Even as a child, something as simple as a game of marbles became a test of my ability to master the problem at hand. When school was out and our chores were done, the boys would sometimes gather in the village courtyard for a game of *golli gundu*.

Carved into the hard-packed dirt were a series of three holes, worn smooth from our many games of *golli*. The objective was to shoot all the glass marbles into the holes, with a finger-flick of another marble, like an American game of billiards. The winner would be rewarded with the honor of rapping a big marble on the losers' knuckles. Whenever I lost, I demanded the harshest punishment. I wanted my knuckles to bleed. And when I won, I would rap those marbles on my friends' knuckles so hard they'd bleed, too. I wasn't cruel. I wanted my friends to be winners as well.

Perhaps it was competition with my older brother, George, that launched my drive to excel. George was better looking; lighter skinned, like my father; stronger; and more athletic than I was. As the eldest child, he was expected to succeed. To be light skinned was considered by many to be preferable to having dark skin, so he was considered not just good-looking but inherently superior. Like any young boy, I looked up to my older brother, who was four years ahead of me. I was dark skinned, like my mother. I was also skinny and had many allergies and never did well in sports, although I did like to play soccer. But I wasn't that good at it. George, on the other hand, was brilliant at soccer, winning many championships as the main goalkeeper. Everybody worshipped him. He was a star in my eyes.

My mother had a friend from high school who became a bishop. When he met George, he was so impressed with this good-looking, charming young boy that he told my mother George would grow up to be the next bishop. He took George under his wing and would send a big white Mercedes-Benz to pick him up and take him to the city. Every time I saw that Mercedes-Benz coming for George, I fumed with resentment. I wasn't getting any attention, and he was being treated like a king!

Given the attention he received, I came to powerfully dislike my brother, but at the same time, I so wanted his attention. Yet no matter how hard I tried, he seemed to take no notice of me, the youngest. He was much nicer to our sister, Gladis. She was right between us in age, two years older than me and two years younger than George. Gladis was serious and quiet but had a strong will.

Because she was a girl, and thus expected to live a quiet life and master the domestic arts, Gladis spent much time on her studies and learning the skills of homemaking and preparing food—which is no small task when it means hauling water from the village well, cooking over an open fire, roasting and pounding the spices, mixing and kneading the rotis and other flat breads by hand. Each meal took hours to prepare, so girls had to start cooking at an early age to help our mothers out.

But as boys, George and I spent much of our time outdoors, often playing, often busy with our chores. Instead of taking me under his wing, however, George would tease me, especially around his friends. Even as small as I was, I vowed to gain his respect. I was determined to earn it and, what's more, to become even more popular and respected than he was.

We lived in the Garden of Eden, at least, that is how the state of Kerala is often described because it is so beautiful and idyllic. It is a land lush with trees bearing coffee, mangoes, passionfruit, coconuts, jackfruit, and cashews—it is impossible to starve amid such aromatic and delicious offerings that God has provided.

In Kerala, iridescent green rice fields circle the simple homes, their long grass undulating in the wind like ocean waves when the harvest is near. Rivers, creeks, and waterfalls and the ever-present rain shroud the hills in a ghostly mist and provide a cooling respite from the enervating heat and humidity. It was always unbearably hot in southern India. Yet the sticky, sweaty heat that so pervades the region is matched by such a heavenly splendor that few would ever want to live anywhere else. Every breath is perfumed with the scent of ripe mangoes and pots of spicy stews simmering over open fires. Peppercorns, cardamom, cinnamon, and nutmeg have not only brought us the most delicious and unique cuisine in all of India, but these same spices have, quite literally, brought us closer to God.

In 1498, the famed explorer Vasco da Gama arrived in my home of Trivandrum in search of spices, gold, silver, silk—and Christians. Spices we had, in abundance—prized sandalwood and the finest cooking spices in the world. And yes, we had gold and silver and the finest silks, even exquisite ivory. As for Christians, while India may be known as a Hindu, Buddhist, and Muslim nation, it is also the home to one of the most ancient centers of Christianity in the world. That history began as far back as AD 52, when the Apostle Thomas came to Kerala and brought the Gospel to our people.

By the time da Gama arrived fifteen hundred years later, one-fifth of the people living in Kerala were Christians, many, like my family, who traced their ancestry back to St. Thomas himself. This was something da Gama did not know.

When he arrived, da Gama asked to meet with the king, and upon meeting him, he told the king, "I come from Portugal and bring blessings from the pope. Have you heard of Christianity?"

The king smiled and told him that there were many Christians living in Kerala, but they lived in the mountains. He promised to arrange an escort so that da Gama could meet these Indian Christians himself.

A few days later, da Gama was indeed escorted to the mountains, where he met with the elders and again announced, "I am Vasco da Gama, and I am a Christian and bring blessings from the pope."

The elders greeted him warmly and said, "We are Christians, too, but who is this pope?"

The pious explorer couldn't imagine Christians who had never heard of the pope, so he set right to correcting that problem!

And that is how our spices brought us closer to God, as da Gama and later Portuguese explorers came for our spices and left us their Catholic church. Kerala now has more Christians than anywhere else in India, and the Catholic tradition has become as much a part of our lives as the land itself. It is this tradition that I was born into, where faith and prayer are inseparable from our daily lives in this Garden of Eden that was my homeland.

Our small village, Murukkumpuzha, is in the district of Trivandrum, the capital city of Kerala in southern India. Trivandrum is built on seven forest-covered hills alongside the sea on the Malabar Coast. I grew to fear the ocean, magnificent yet terrifying in its vast power. But it was the ocean that gave us life, bringing us the freshest, tastiest fish so that no one, no matter how poor, would ever go hungry.

Each morning the fishmonger would walk through the village with a large basket balanced on his head, calling *meen, meen, meen*—the Malayalam word for fish. Once or twice a week when my mother heard this sound, she would stop whatever she was doing and follow the call of the fishmonger to see what he had to offer that day.

I would often join my mother, standing close to her legs, small and timid yet excited to know that we would have fresh fish—possibly even my favorite curried fish stew—that night. She would gather around the fishmonger with the other women in the village, and when it was her turn, she would inspect the fish, so fresh the gills might still be beating. She made sure that the eyes were bright, the gills red, the flesh firm, the catch of the day not too bony. Once satisfied, she began her bargaining.

"How much for this one?" she would ask the fishmonger, pointing to a particularly nice fish.

"Ten rupees," he might say, or some other amount my mother had no intention of paying and he had no expectation of receiving.

"No, five rupees," she'd counter, her voice firm but kind.

"Okay, I will sell you this fish for seven rupees," the fishmonger would respond, and both would smile.

"Okay, I will buy it," she'd finally decide, and hand the coins to the fishmonger as he wrapped our fish in banana leaves and offered it to me to carry. We had little money, so every purchase of fresh fish or shellfish would be a blessing from God, no matter how often we ate it.

Another blessing from God I would later come to understand was the lesson my mother was teaching me in how to be wise with money and how not to take any meal for granted, a lesson that has lasted me a lifetime.

The fish from the ocean came at a cost to our village, however, a cost much higher than rupees. Every year a certain number of men would sail out to the ocean to bring back a good catch, and every year a certain number would never return. We learned early on to respect the sea, which took so many lives yet gave us life.

My mother so feared losing me to those waters that she forbade me from playing in the ocean, and for that reason, I never learned to swim. I was her youngest, and she couldn't bear to lose me, and because I was such a small and skinny child, the chances were great that she would. I would watch as the other children played in the ocean and rivers and lakes, while I remained on shore or waded only a few feet out, knowing that the waters were for others to play in. But I had different pursuits, so I did not dwell on what I could not do. Instead, I focused on the many things I could do, and do better than most.

One of my many chores would be to help dry the fish, which we spread on grass mats laid along the street, where they would dry in the sun to be stored in our homes for future meals. The briny, salty smell of the sea that filled our homes and village was thus a constant reminder of the benevolence of God, a smell softened by the fruity aroma of ripe mangoes and stores of cinnamon and cardamom that were so plentiful.

Another chore was guarding the rice fields from the birds. The birds would descend on the ripening rice grains, and if we didn't scare them away with our slingshots, they'd devour the whole crop. To protect the fields, after school all the boys would head to the rice fields and shoot stones at the pesky thieves. I got pretty good at it and could spot a bird from a hectare away and hit it in an instant.

We had chickens, of course, but they pretty much took care of themselves, wandering around the village clucking and pecking as if they were gossiping neighbors without a care in the world. We had cows, too, and one of my chores was to pasture the cattle. I wasn't allowed to milk the cows, which was fine with me, as that was an early-morning chore, and a rather dangerous one at that. If you didn't pull on the teat just right, or the cow was simply in a bad mood, it would kick, and not only could that cause quite an injury, but it would almost always knock over the pail and send the milk flying, which we could ill afford. Fortunately, we hired a man to do the early-morning milking, so that task didn't fall to me or to George.

After scaring away the birds, George and I would have a snack, maybe a spicy *dosha* or deep-fried banana chips. Then we'd take the cows out to pasture so they could eat. By this time, it would be evening, and each day it took longer and longer because we had to take them farther and farther out to find grass that they hadn't already devoured. Then we'd bring them home and shower with a bucket pulled up from the well and go inside and do our homework.

I whizzed through my homework as if every assignment were another goal to achieve. I absolutely loved going to school, and it came as naturally to me as sports came to George. I had a keen mind and memory. Whatever it was—reading, math, Malayalam, Hindi, or English—I absorbed it as readily as I absorbed the sun and the heat. But for George, academics were a challenge. He was a social charmer and an impressive athlete, but he struggled with his schoolwork. Fortunately for me, his struggle proved to be my opportunity.

We went to school together or sometimes with other kids from the village. We left early in the morning, our feet bare, crossing the rice fields by walking along the narrow bunds, which were the mounds of mud that divided the paddies and held the muddy water. They could be slippery and were usually no wider than a foot across, and we often slipped. The paddies weren't deep, but they were filled with cow dung, parasites, leeches, and snakes, so we did our best to hurry along and not slip.

Once we reached the ends of the rice fields, there was another walkway of about a quarter mile before we reached the main road where the cars and buses passed. There we walked along the road for about a mile until we reached the school by 9:00 a.m. It was a long trek to school, but we all did it together, so it was always enjoyable.

While doing homework at home, I sat behind George and could see his work, so I knew when he needed help. He had a tough time in most of his subjects, not because he wasn't smart, but because he wasn't book smart. But I was both, so I'd help him with the answers, as well as with his homework, and pretty soon he stopped teasing me and came to respect me. And as he respected me, I stopped resenting him. It wasn't long before George became a really nice guy, and I was proud to be his younger brother.

I also came to see that I enjoyed helping people with their school-work and, more importantly, that I had a valuable skill. Growing up as poor as we were, having anything of value was a step out of poverty, so I worked hard to master my studies, even when I didn't need to work very hard at it. I'd been blessed with a good mind, something my family recognized right from the start.

Now, these years that I recall here were over half a century ago, not long after India first gained its independence from Great Britain in 1947. Trivandrum has since burst into modernity with endless ribbons of speeding roads and buildings at the capital city.

Trivandrum has advanced so remarkably since I was a child that it has now become one of the technology hubs for southern India and a center of intellectual and scientific acclaim. But I was not born into this modern world. I was born in 1951, in the home of my grandparents, my mother assisted not by a doctor but a midwife, just as she'd been with the two children she bore before me. And it was in that home that my destiny was shaped.

When I was born, my grandfather, a very wise man and somewhat a mystic, perceived that there was something special about me. When shortly after my birth an Indian astrologer forecast that I would become a powerful man, a detriment to my enemies, and a blessing to my friends and family, my grandfather said, "One man can change the history of the world, good or bad. And I want this child to do that." And that is why he chose for me the name he felt most noble and fitting—Lenin. This name, however seemingly incongruous with the trajectory of my life, was not chosen for its ideology but for its power. Let me explain.

As India struggled for its independence from the British in the late 1940s, my grandfather, a true intellectual who was well read and kept current in world affairs, had come to know many Russians. He would send them Indian movies and other coveted gifts, and in return, they sent him vodka and books and other coveted Russian goods. My grandfather became intrigued by the success of the Russian Revolution. Many Indians in Kerala were active in the Communist Party, and in 1957, they would elect one of the world's first elected communist governments, an understandable direction considering the long history of outsiders controlling our country and seizing our land and resources for their own gain, a topic to which I'll return.

My grandfather had become a wealthy landowner, and he would later denounce communism, but at that time he viewed communism as the just response to a society that had for too long deprived people of the basic necessities of life—food, clothing, and housing. Workers had been treated brutally in Czarist Russia, and as a Christian who cared that everyone be treated with dignity and respect, he found much to admire in the new leaders of the Soviet Union, then in its adolescence. And thus, in christening me with the name Lenin, my grandfather committed to ensuring my future would, like that of the Soviet leader Vladimir Lenin, be a great one.

But I am getting ahead of myself. Let me first tell you about my family, my childhood, and why I was so eager to leave this Garden of Eden. As you will see, it is not because I sought to leave my family. No, not at all. It was instead my destiny that I leave Kerala for both myself and for my family—and follow in the path God laid before me, on a journey that has brought riches unimaginable to a small village boy growing up so far from the world I now inhabit. Here is my story.

❧ CHAPTER 2 ❧

Holding Court
on the Veranda

My grandparents were extraordinary people, my grandfather especially. I remember him as a very tall and slim man with thick silver hair and deep penetrating eyes. He dressed in the traditional Indian style of long loose shirts and exquisite slippers or shoes. With every step he took, he walked straight and tall and with great pride, always carrying an expensive walking stick with a gold-plated handle. Not that he needed the stick for support. It was just his way of showing his authority, an authority he had well earned.

It was he who was my greatest influence as I grew, and I cannot tell the story of my life without telling the story of my grandfather, Maria John Lopez. He was born sometime in the late nineteenth century, an only child whose mother died when he was young. As an only child, her property, which was vast, had passed to him, making him a large landowner at a young age. His father remarried but had no children with his second wife, who raised my grandfather as her own. When they died, large landowners themselves, their property also passed to their only child. Thus it was that my grandfather entered life as a young man with a great deal of land. He was also a well-educated Christian, spoke

English, and possessed a keen business sense, all qualities that ensured he was well respected and his future secure.

He married another Christian, Catharina, my grandmother, and over the next several years they had six children, four boys and two girls. The second child was my mother, Philomena Lopez, and the third was her sister, my aunt Lourdes. Fourth was Freddy and fifth was Augustine. Sixth came Christopher.

The eldest, Sonny, was exceptionally bright. He became an engineer and moved to Kuala Lumpur, where he helped develop the infrastructure for the city of Singapore. He was wildly successful, but he never came back, marrying a woman from Singapore and raising their three children there.

Perhaps it was the stories of my uncle Sonny that first planted in me the voyager seeds—hearing the tales of this adventurous man who traveled halfway around the world to find riches and acclaim excited me with possibilities far beyond the idyllic but provincial world in which I grew. Or perhaps it was the spirit of my mother, which so filled me with an unshakable belief in myself and in my destiny, that set me on my path.

At the time of my grandparents' marriage, India was under the rule of King George V, a rather dull and conventional monarch yet one whose visit to India nearly a decade before had brought great fanfare to the nation. But by the time my mother was born in 1920, a rising anti-colonialist nationalist from western India by the name of Mahatma Gandhi was making a name for himself advocating the nonviolent overthrow of the British colonial forces, which had ruled our country since the late eighteenth century. So it was that my mother was born into these turbulent times, where the future for landlords like my grandfather was uncertain and the need for faith all the more pressing.

As the firstborn daughter, my mother became my grandfather's favorite, and no doubt my grandmother's as well. They treasured her and were devoted to ensuring she was protected. She was taught to read and write and early on was introduced to the Christian rituals and traditions, which sparked in her an immediate and lifelong devotion to prayer and faith.

While it was uncommon for girls to go to university in those days, my grandparents made sure that Philomena had a high school education and learned to speak English. She did so, but it was her faith that would prove to be her greatest virtue and strength. She spent her days in prayer, reciting the Rosary, memorizing the Gospel. She went to church every day, where she discussed the Gospel with the priest. As she reached the end of her studies, she knew what she wanted to do with her life.

"Father," she told him, "I am almost of age, and I know what I must do with my life. I want to devote my life to Christ, and to do that, I would like to take my vows and become a nun."

Her decision surprised nobody, because since she was a child, Philomena's passion was for God and the Church. But my grandfather would not agree.

"No, Philomena," he told her. "That is not your destiny, my child. You will marry and have children." His mind was made up—as the eldest daughter, she was not destined to sequester herself inside a convent, but to pass on the gifts that God had blessed our family with by continuing our lineage.

She knew there was no point in challenging his decision, as a father's will could not be questioned. Although my mother was heartbroken to be told she could not be a nun, she accepted her destiny, but she was determined to remain devoted to Christ.

As my grandfather's landholdings grew and he was able to collect rent and increase his wealth, he purchased a post office, an acquisition that positioned him well in the community. And because her English skills were good, after my mother finished school, my grandfather told her she was to become the postmistress, which gave her a respected status. He understood that it was important for her to both be respected and gain professional experience, so that she could marry well and find her place in society.

My mother enjoyed the work, and she excelled at her position. What's more, she met many people and still had time for her devotions and prayers. Rather than resent my grandfather for not permitting her to become a nun, she came to realize that a secular life could still be a life of devotion and a life of service.

When it became time to find a respected man for my mother to marry, she again knew that while she had a voice, she did not have the ultimate choice. At that time in India, who one married was determined by the bride's and groom's parents, not the bride and groom themselves. My grandparents had learned of a bright, university-educated man named Joseph Peter. Joseph Peter was ten years my mother's senior, and he worked in the big city of Bombay, now known as Mumbai.

In the course of his work, my father interacted with people from across India, as well as all over the world, particularly the British. He came from a respected family in Kundara, a small town in Kerala north of our village. He was the oldest in a family of nine children and admired by both his family and his community. It was expected that given his English skills, education, intellectual interests, as well as his good looks, Joseph Peter would be a fine match for Philomena Lopez. And given that she was the eldest daughter of the esteemed Maria John Lopez, and a beautiful woman at that, Philomena Lopez was a bride worthy of only a man of good birth and prospect. Thus it was that shortly before their wedding, my mother and my father met for the first time. Fortunately, they were both pleased with the match their parents had made, and the two were promptly married.

Now, before I go any further, I must explain something unique about Kerala culture. We are a matrilineal society, which means that while we take our father's name, we trace our lineage through our mothers, a practice that gives women much greater status and rights than is found in many societies. This is not to say that men are not important. Far from it. Men are the patriarchs of the home and community in Kerala, but a man has equal responsibility to his own biological children and to his sisters' children. That meant that while my father would care for us and love us and provide for us financially, his equal responsibility would be to his sisters' children, of which there were several.

It was my mother's brothers who would have the greatest roles in my life and my siblings' lives. Sonny was the eldest brother, but as I've noted, he had established a wholly unconventional but respected life in a land far away. In the early part of the twentieth century, sending money home from Singapore to India was no simple task. With Sonny gone, it would be my uncle Augustine who would play the role of father figure in my life as I grew up. But again, I am getting ahead of myself and do not want to bore you with a lesson in Indian kinship systems.

The point I wish to press upon you is that my father's responsibilities were not those one would expect of an American father in the twenty-first century. It was up to him to equally provide for his sisters and their children, as well as care for our family once his own sisters were taken care of.

My father was the oldest of all the siblings, with two sisters, Mary and Clara, and brothers, from oldest to youngest, Alphonse, Sebastian, Isaac, Henry, and Johnson.

With such responsibility to his family pressing upon my father, it was necessary that he make a good living. Fortunately, it was during this time that educated Indians who spoke English were in great demand in the oil-producing country of Yemen, so it was no surprise that my father accepted a coveted position with British Petroleum in Aden, a port city in Yemen under British control. With his absence, my mother remained living with her parents for the first four years of my life.

Of course, I do not remember these days because I was so small, but by about the time I was four years old, my mother and father had built a small home in the village of Murukkumpuzha, about an hour and a half bus ride away from the capital city of Trivandrum. My father continued to work in Yemen, however, returning for one month each year. While he made a good deal of money, he supported his sisters' children, was generous with all his friends, and spent a great deal as well on whoever needed help. As a result, he did not send us much money.

Because of my father's obligations as well as his spending habits, my mother cared for her three children on her own, and though we struggled economically, she never complained. Instead, she focused on all the blessings God had bestowed upon her and faced each day with a calm and loving smile.

Nonetheless, it was difficult for my mother. Consequently, after about a year, when I was five years old, and as my mother struggled to manage her three children all by herself, my grandfather proposed a solution. He explained to her that he recognized in me certain gifts that his many other grandchildren had not demonstrated. Desiring to build upon those traits, he determined that I would be his successor as patriarch of the family, and to prepare me for that role, I was to live with him.

My mother adored me and did not want to give me up, but she could see that this arrangement would be the best for everyone. She made the difficult decision to send me to my grandparents, where I would live under their care. I remember going to their home for what I thought was a short visit, and while I was excited to visit my grandmother and grandfather, when it became time for my mother to leave and return to the village, I was heartbroken that she would not let me return with her. I could not understand why she would abandon me like that, and knowing that my brother and sister remained with her, I felt as if she preferred them to me. In the mind of a five-year-old, there are few alternative explanations, and so it was that I wept and longed for my mother's return.

It hadn't occurred to me when my mother left me at my grandparents' home that I would be staying there for long. At first I had assumed she would be back in a few days, and when she did not return, I assumed she'd return in a few weeks. But gradually, as the weeks passed and she didn't return and school began, I grew to accept my new life. It was certainly a much more comfortable life. They lived in a grand home, on two or three acres of land. The home itself had a big patio covered with broad banana leaves to keep out the rain, where my grandparents entertained visitors and my grandfather often held court with the many people who sought him out. There were many rooms, all beautifully furnished, and I had my own bedroom all to myself. It was a princely life, even if I did miss my mother terribly.

As I settled into my new life, however, the longing I felt for my mother was soon replaced with happiness as I became the center of my loving grandparents' attention. They showered me with love and attention, and it wasn't long before I would find myself hiding whenever my mother came to visit, which she did every couple of months or so. Whether it was because I was angry with her for abandoning me or I just didn't want to leave once settled into this new life, I am not sure, for how can one recall accurately the thoughts and emotions one feels at such a tender age? But my memory of hiding from my mother is clear, as she would arrive to take me back home for a weekend or a week, and I would run away and hide. I just didn't want to go. I had grown so close to my grandparents, especially my grandfather, that I no longer wanted to return home. His home had become my home, and I was thriving in that environment.

He played the fiddle beautifully and filled the house with music, just as my grandmother filled the home with her delicious seafood stews and other dishes from her ancestral Portugal and southern India. To this day, I remember those times as some of the happiest I've ever known, and the joy I felt in the company of my grandfather is a joy that has lasted me throughout my life.

Men and women ate separately back then, and men and boys were always served first. I was so proud when my grandfather would ask me to sit next to him and offer me the best food at the table, even before his own two sons had taken theirs. My uncles did not mind, though, for they adored me as well.

The food my grandmother prepared was always delicious—fresh fish, chicken, beef, pork—we ate it all. As for what she and my aunts ate, I do not know, as the women ate in a separate room. They may have had less public power than men at that time, but their informal power was great. After all, they were the ones who decided what it was we ate, and for all I know, they ate much grander meals than we did!

I quickly discovered how to maximize every opportunity with my adoring grandfather. Every time he gave me one inch, I took a foot. If he asked me to sit near him, I wiggled even closer to him. If he ate one piece of good food, I ate two pieces. I enjoyed every minute of it, and being the youngest in the family, I got away with it. And as I got away with it, I realized that there was no reason not to. By watching my grandfather, I was coming to learn that the path to success was in many ways just in the taking. So I fully intended to take as much as life would offer me, just as long as I didn't deprive anyone in the process.

Watching my grandfather became a fascination. I was particularly fascinated by how others responded to him. My grandfather's skills as a mediator were widely known, and it wasn't uncommon that in the evening the front parlor would become busy with people who had come to him to resolve some dispute or problem. Rather than go to a judge when they had a problem, they would come to him because they so respected his wisdom. He would invite the opposing parties to sit on the veranda in the open air overlooking his vast estate, as he paced up and down in the courtyard, listening to their differing perspectives and concerns. The heat would be nearly unbearable, but it never detracted from their rapt attention as he spoke.

"I think you are right," he would say to one or both parties after hearing them plead their case. "But this is what we are going to do." He would then propose a solution, and they would inevitably agree that his decision was a just and wise one, and everyone would leave satisfied that they had reached an agreement.

As I sat at his feet in the awful heat, I marveled at how confidently and wisely he responded to those who came to him for counsel. While the details of whatever problem was being discussed were far too complicated for my young mind to fully understand, as I paid attention to their interactions I came to see that for every problem there is a solution, and by finding that solution, great progress can be made. While I could not have foreseen it at the time, it was by appreciating that fundamental principle that I was able to succeed even when everything appeared to be stacked against me.

My grandfather took it upon himself to nurture me toward success at an early age, and one of the things I loved to do was dress up. I especially liked dressing up as a doctor, because doctors were educated and important. So I would put on a white jacket, sling something around my neck like a stethoscope, and announce, "I'm a doctor today!" My grandfather was pleased with this activity, and every day he would ask me, "Who are you going to be today?" or "What important person are you going to be today?"

I recognized quickly that my grandfather wanted me to be someone important, so I had to learn who all the important people were. Soon I was dressing up as Gandhi or Churchill or whoever was important and in the news. By dressing up and pretending to be these important people, I soon began to see myself as an important person, and I so wanted to make my grandfather proud. I knew then, even at the age of five, that someday I would be a real doctor, and more than that, an important person to my people.

After living with my grandfather for a year, it was time for me to return to my mother. I had visited her often during my stay with my grandparents, but it was time for me to start another year of school, and my mother missed me terribly. I did not want to leave my grandfather's house, but I had friends in my village and I missed my mother. So I returned to my mother and resumed the busy life of chores and outdoor play, though for the next several years, until I was about ten years old, I moved back and forth between their two homes.

I hadn't been back at my mother's very long before I got into trouble. At the end of the rice paddies there was a field with a pond where the Hindus had placed a statue of one of their gods and constructed a shrine, where they would go to worship. They revered snakes, which they believed were devotees of their gods, and prohibited killing them. Consequently, the pond was teeming with poisonous snakes, so not many people took a dip there.

Since I couldn't swim and it was so infested with deadly snakes, I was not allowed to go there. But one afternoon around five o'clock, after school had let out, some of us decided to go there. I knew I wasn't supposed to, but I wanted to play with the older boys, so I did go, and walked into the pond and splashed around.

I was terribly afraid of snakes, which we would see slithering all over the place near our home. They were especially difficult to see at dusk, or in the night, so to scare them off we would dry coconut leaves in the sun, bind the dried leaves to long sticks, and set them on fire. These burning torches would scare away the cobras and small pythons, but the snakes always remained a constant presence in our lives. And as we never wore shoes, because they simply weren't available and wearing shoes or even sandals is next to impossible when passing through rice paddies, we were continually stepping on snakes as we walked through the village or in the courtyards.

The snakes were all over the place, in the rice paddies and ponds, at the base of the trees, just everywhere, including poisonous cobras, vipers, and pythons. My brother didn't mind them—lots of kids didn't—but I just hated them. Yet I was so overcome by the excitement of playing at the pond that I set my fear aside and walked barefoot into the dark water.

I hadn't been in the pond long before I saw a snake. I couldn't tell what kind it was, but just as I turned to get away, I felt the most piercing pain in my butt. I got out of the water grabbing my butt. The boys laughed uproariously while I ran around howling in pain. I didn't know if it was a leech or a snake, but it hurt like hell, and when I checked, I saw two distinct fang marks that began bleeding profusely. Once they saw the fang marks, the boys stopped laughing and saw that the situation was serious. They thought I was going to die because it was bleeding so badly.

Even though I knew I would get into big trouble when my mother found out I'd gone to the pond, I had no choice but to tell her. I ran home as fast as I could, crying my heart out all the way, terrified that the snake had been a poisonous one and I would die.

My mom was furious that I'd gone to the pond, but she didn't have time to focus on her anger—she knew I was suffering already. Once she examined the bite, however, she assured me it was not from a poisonous snake and I wouldn't have to go to the hospital. But the bleeding continued for the rest of the afternoon and nearly until bedtime. I learned my lesson and stayed clear of the pond from that day forward.

Life with my mother was good, though the house was much smaller than my grandfather's. Our house was a colorful and simple but traditional thatch-covered one made of clay, perched on a hill and quite isolated from other homes. Though humble, it was a nice home, painted yellow with red and blue trim and surrounded by mango, coconut, and cashew trees. I especially liked the veranda, where we could sit and enjoy the lovely view of the trees, as well as all the spices and vegetables that grew around our home—black pepper, red and green peppers, ginger, okra, yucca. We never went hungry.

And on each side of the veranda was a room. In one room we stored our rice. The room itself was elevated, to keep the rats out, and inside was a big storage container that took up most of the space. On the other side of the veranda was where my parents slept, though most often it was just my mom, as my father worked in Yemen. Inside the house was one big area with a table, where we ate and I studied, our kitchen, and the bedroom where I slept with my brother and sister. We had two wooden pallets built off the floor, though often we slept right on the floor. It was a simple home, but it was filled with color, the aroma of good food cooking throughout the day, and most of all, it was a home filled with a lot of love.

There were big windows in the house overlooking the mango trees, and beyond the trees was a pathway leading to the paddy fields that I'd cross to get to school, or where I worked chasing away the birds and the women worked planting and threshing the rice.

The work there was harder and the food not quite as good but still tasty. But my mother always got the rice flour and lentils prepared each evening so in the mornings it would be ready to be cooked for break-fast. We always had a good breakfast and fresh milk, and she always packed me a good but simple lunch to take to school, usually some veg-etables or *dosha* or fish wrapped in banana leaves that I would unwrap and eat with my hands, which is how we always ate in India.

As I've said, I loved school and loved studying, and I found the most perfect place to study far from any interruption. There was a beautiful cashew tree near our house, which had broad limbs and was easy to climb. I could sit in that tree for hours, just studying, or gazing at the world through the magical mosaic of leaves that fell like a canopy around me. There was absolute peace in that tree, and no matter how much chaos there was at home, I could always find sanctuary there.

Most of the chaos came just once a year, however, with the annual arrival of my father. One month out of the year my father returned home, and going to the railway station to meet him was a big hoopla. I was always excited to see my father. We all were.

Unfortunately, although I loved him dearly and he was a good man, my father had developed a drinking problem in Yemen, and he brought that problem home to us. He wasn't too bad when I was very young, but his drinking got progressively worse, and by the time I was around eight years old, once he got good and drunk, his temper would soar. He particularly took his anger out on my brother, George.

If George's grades weren't good, he would be in for it with our dad. It was only later that we learned that George suffered from dyslexia, but back then no one knew what dyslexia was. They just thought he wasn't very smart. But I realized that if George did well in his studies, my father wouldn't be angry, so I did my best to help George with his exams.

My father was very hard on George, and I'm not sure why. Maybe because George was the eldest son, and my father wanted him to be perfect. He was constantly correcting George, even to the point of telling him how to sleep. George would sleep on his back, but my father insisted he had to sleep on his side and would wake him at night and berate him for not sleeping properly. So whenever my father was home, I made sure to turn George onto his side while he slept so that my father would not wake him up.

As I relate these stories, I want to emphasize that my father was, first and foremost, a nice man, one of the kindest men I ever knew. But alcohol was his demon, and as children of alcoholics realize early on, I learned how to keep my father happy and keep peace in the house any way that I could. But sometimes his demon was so great it proved far beyond my control.

One night, when I was eight years old, I woke at 3:00 a.m. to the most horrifying scene. Hearing the cries of my mother, I peered out the window and saw my father running around outside our small house stark naked, carrying a giant, burning torch made of dried coconut husks as he raged at my mother. I was terrified he was going to burn the house down, and us along with it.

Fortunately, my mother said something, and he calmed right down as if she'd tranquilized him with her words. My mother had an amazing serenity about her at all times, and this was one time when her inner peace worked its magic on my father's internal tempest. What it was that had set him off that night, I don't know. He'd probably come home from the bar quite late and my mother had told him that was not acceptable or some such thing. But whatever it was, seeing him in that state terrified us all, and we were eager to have our home back to its normal state when he left that year.

Although I was young, I understood that my father had a problem he couldn't control. As I grew older, I came to realize he worked so hard in Yemen, where there were so few opportunities to do anything other than work, that the workers were rewarded with endless alcohol to keep them pacified. In my father's case, however, the alcohol did quite the opposite, and as the years went on, his addiction saddled him with a heavy heart because he could not quit it.

He also became reckless with his money, buying drinks for his friends, becoming overly generous once he'd had too much to drink, and even losing it as it fell from his pockets. I remember seeing my mother following him, picking up the coins that fell from his pockets as he staggered home. He had little to send us as a result, and we lived in virtual poverty, something I vowed I would overcome so that I could help my family as soon as I was able.

Through all these difficult times, my mother never said a harsh word about my father and never once complained of the difficult life she led. "Your father is a good man," she would say, or, "Your father is a nice man. Be grateful." She never spoke ill of him, no matter how hard her life had become. She understood my father's drinking was a weakness he could not control, but she loved and admired him for the man he was beyond the drink. And she accepted that while she may not have been a wealthy woman and had a life of hard work and little material comfort, she was blessed beyond imagining. Her life of faith and prayer had given her a perspective and purpose that made such difficulties unimportant.

Watching her face shine with joy when she spoke of God or rest in such a peaceful expression when she said her Rosary struck a magical note inside me as well. But when she announced that in addition to going to church on Saturdays and Sundays, I would be joining her every Tuesday evening for a visit to St. Anthony's Shrine, I was not at all happy. By that time, because I was showing such promise in school, I was attending before-school lessons and after-school lessons and even going to school through the summer. I'd been placed on a fast track in school that kept me so busy, I couldn't imagine adding yet another obligation, even if it was just once a week. But my mother was adamant I had to go.

"Lenny," she admonished me, "you must be prepared to die for your faith."

I did not want to die, and young as I was, I could not imagine why she wanted me to do so. What I did not realize at the time, but she clearly did, was that she was not preparing me to die, but to live, and that the experience would transform me and set me on my future path.

⮐ CHAPTER 3 ⮎

In the Glow
of St. Anthony's Shrine

St. Anthony's Shrine radiated serenity and love. Small but spacious, its courtyard cooled by the shade of cashew trees, I immediately felt relaxed. We stepped inside the open-air shrine, the calming aroma of burning candles warming my soul. It was a humble shrine, and though not very colorful, it felt comforting.

A statue of St. Anthony stood behind a column where they kept the sacrament, and before the statue were the candles, which, for a small offering, the faithful could light. There were no walls, so when it was raining we would get wet, but no one seemed to mind. Despite my initial reluctance, I soon found that the shrine offered a peaceful yet joyful respite from the chaos of my young life.

I was still a child, just eight years old or so, yet already I felt such a heavy burden of responsibility on me. I knew that all the favor I received from my family came with a cost—I was expected to succeed, to become an important person, and my family had impressed upon me that God had gifted me with a unique mind. Indeed, I knew I was smart, smarter than any others I knew. I needed only to scan a page of words and they were imprinted in my memory. I needed only to hear a problem once to discern a solution. Just as my grandfather had been gifted with an unparalleled wisdom, so did I feel that I had received a gift that I could not waste, and I was frequently reminded of this responsibility before me. What's more, the faster my mind worked, the faster my program of study accelerated until I was studying nearly around the clock, which, as much as I loved my schoolwork, became a constant source of stress.

Other burdens pressed upon me, adding to my sense that my family depended on me to make something special of myself. Watching my brother struggle with his studies, I continued to help him succeed. My mother struggled with raising our family alone with little money, since my father was in Yemen most of the year. And when he returned, his drinking brought fear and chaos to our home—yet, at the same time, when he would leave to return to Yemen, I would be heartbroken, for I loved my father dearly. I worried for him as I saw him struggle with his addiction to the whiskey, which transformed him as if an evil spirit had overpowered him. Through it all, I was shuttled back and forth between my grandparents' home and my own home, and as much as I loved being in both places, the constant back-and-forth while keeping up with my studies intensified my stress.

Added to all these personal challenges for such a young boy, I was somewhat of an outcast in my own country. As Christians we were a minority even in Kerala, and with that came a certain level of teasing and ostracizing that, while not too harsh, compounded my anxiety. Yet it was through Christianity that I found respite from my social alienation, as the weekly trips to St. Anthony's soon transformed from a burden to a grace.

A small group gathered every Tuesday evening to light candles and say the full Rosary. I would watch as my mother and several other women would light candles together and, kneeling upon the cement floor, pray for their special intentions. I found that in joining them in this prayer, I felt peace. As time passed, this small congregation grew larger, bringing an even greater anchor to my faith and stimulating my spirit to new heights. I am sure I did not articulate the sensation in quite that way at that young age, but I felt an excitement as I anticipated our trips to the shrine each week and a comforting inner calm that came over me once we got there.

Because we met on Tuesdays, my mother would say the Sorrowful Mysteries as she said the Rosary, meditating on the sorrows of Jesus Christ. Each Mystery was to be said on a different day, and listening to her rapt in concentration on the sufferings of Christ, I felt my own sufferings lift. My mother taught me that the Rosary could become a powerful weapon against suffering, helping me to see that through prayer and contemplation, any hardship could be overcome. For a boy struggling with so many burdens, such assurance was profound—I steadily gained a powerful faith that no matter what problems might beset me, I would be protected by the Lord Jesus Christ and would find my way if only I had faith.

My mother was the proof of this simple precept. She endured so much hardship as she raised us in our small home, with neither electricity nor running water and a husband she saw only a month out of the year—and often intoxicated at that. Yet she never complained, never once cursed her fate. She did not hesitate to speak her mind, as she was a strong woman, yet she never had a bad word for anyone. Her faith in the Lord Jesus Christ had infused in her a radiance that few in this world possess. Each week when we would walk the long route to St. Anthony's, no matter how poor she was, my mother always brought an offering to give to the Saint, and in return she would ask for blessings—and most times those blessings she requested were for me.

Her favorite prayer, however, was the Angelus, which she devotedly recited in Latin three times a day, at 6:00 a.m., again at noon, and again at 6:00 p.m.

> *Angelus Domini nuntiavit Mariæ,*
>
> *Et concepit de Spiritu Sancto.*
>
> *Ave Maria, gratia plena, Dominus tecum.*

Benedicta tu in mulieribus, et benedictus fructus ventris tui, Iesus.

The angel of the Lord declared unto Mary

And she conceived of the Holy Spirit

Hail Mary, full of grace, the Lord is with thee: blessed art thou amongst women, and blessed is the Fruit of thy womb, Jesus.

After the prayers, she would distribute freshly baked bread rolls and bananas to the poor, who had even less than we had.

"But, Mama," I would protest when I saw her pocket a few coins to take to the shrine or fill a basket with bread and bananas. "We need that for ourselves. We don't have enough to give away."

"But we do have enough, my son," she would answer. "Giving to others is our way of thanking St. Anthony for the favors we've received when he has answered our prayers."

I would nod, contemplating that simple truth, as I helped her pass out the rolls and bananas. We had so little, yet my mother was right. We had been blessed with all that we needed.

Still, I wanted more, and I knew in my heart that when I grew up, I would have an abundance of favor. But to attain that abundance, I would need faith.

It was about this same time that my spirit was opening up to God, that my mind was opening up to the world. With my uncle in Singapore and my father in Yemen, I was already aware that there was a much greater world beyond Kerala. India had attained independence a few years before I was born, yet the influence of the British in our country was still great. I pondered how it could be that these British colonialists could come into our country of nearly six hundred million and conquer it so easily.

At one point there were fifteen thousand Indians for every British person in India. Given how we outnumbered them, something must be wrong with us, I reasoned. Was it that we were inherently weak? I wondered. What was it about these foreigners that gave them such power? I pondered this question as I grappled to understand the world while growing up in the wake of foreign occupation.

Fortunately, my father had given us a small battery-operated transistor radio, which quickly became a portal into this unknown world. We had no electricity, of course, so we had never watched television. But with that small radio, I could turn the dial, listening to the static broken by bits of sound, often indiscernible, but every now and then a station would come in clearly, and I could listen for hours. One station that I could always rely on played Voice of America, and listening to it changed my world.

That little radio became my best friend, and every evening I would go out to my cashew tree, climb onto my favorite limb, and tune into the Voice of America. I couldn't get enough of this America. America was a magical country, I came to believe, and learning about it opened up my view of the world. As it did so, I became less interested in local politics and what was happening in the rest of India and who was ruling what and who was fighting over this or that. In its place, I became fascinated by what was happening outside our country, and more importantly, what was happening in America as its economy and technology soared in the years following the Second World War. Sitting in my cashew tree listening to Voice of America, I was becoming a global citizen—and I wanted to learn more.

As good fortune would have it, my father had invited us to spend a year with him in Aden, Yemen. I had never traveled farther than my grandfather's home, so the opportunity to sail across the Arabian Sea and live with my father for the entire year was absolutely thrilling. I had never even seen a big boat before, much less been on one, and this one was an enormous ship—it was bigger than anything I'd ever seen before. Boarding that ship was like stepping into another world, as if entering the portal of a magnificent floating palace. Day after day, we all stood by the window and watched the sea as it took us farther away from land—and farther away from India. My mind and spirit were so alive and excited to be transported across such vast waters, knowing they were taking us to an exotic world where not even the words people spoke would be familiar.

It was a wonderful trip, and we had a good life there. Because my father was working all day, he did not drink much, and when he was not drinking, he was a very nice man, so kind and loving, and a very social person, as well. Because of his position managing the central supply for the workers at British Petroleum, he had a great deal of influence—he could pretty much get anyone anything. That made him quite popular, and his popularity, along with his English skills, enabled him to get membership with the British expatriate club—in fact, he was the only Indian admitted to the club.

Every weekend we would go to the club and play card games or whatever activities they had for the kids. They had many costume parties, and we would sometimes dress up in costumes and just have a good time. I loved seeing my mother and father dressed up and enjoying their time together. Living in Yemen that year was the first time we had really lived like a family, with both my parents together.

The house my father lived in was a company home, owned by British Petroleum. The house was very large, quite nice, and for the first time I lived in a home with electricity and running water. But sandstorms blew the desert sands so fiercely that some days half the house would be covered in a layer of sand, which was most unpleasant. Yet the near weekly occurrence was a minor inconvenience given the many blessings the trip offered.

Among those blessings was living among people from all over the world. There were Filipinos, Eastern Europeans, Pakistanis. I played with them all, though I avoided many of the local Yemeni kids because I did not quite care for them—many were so wealthy and spoiled that they had no motivation to do anything at all. They didn't even go to school. I continued to study from sunrise to sunset, and while we were homeschooled during this period, it wasn't much of an adjustment for me because I was already self-driven when it came to academics. My brother and sister worked with tutors primarily, but I preferred to work alone, poring through my textbooks as if they were entertaining comic books—every page brought a new discovery. I even picked up some Arabic while I was there.

There were two motivations driving me during this time. The first was that I had already developed a fear of poverty. My fear did not arise from our own poverty. Though we were certainly poor in India, I had come to see that there were many people far more poor than we were, and I was determined I would never end up in such a state. While living with my father, I was also discovering a world of wealth in Yemen, and a much more comfortable lifestyle. I saw no reason why I should not live in such comfort myself, and I knew that the only way that could be possible would be through my education.

The other motivation that kept me so keenly focused on my studies was my thirst for knowledge. Books brought an entirely new world into my life, a world that extended far beyond Kerala, and I soaked up every page. Through books, and the knowledge they imparted, the world became so much larger, and in turn, so did I. That year in Yemen became a year of discovery that had introduced me to new people, new cultures, and an intensive course of self-study that ignited my spirit as it had never been before.

But alas, that remarkable year eventually came to an end. I did not want to return to India, but it was not up to me, and I accepted that it was time to leave my father, with whom I'd grown much closer. But as we sailed back across the Arabian Sea, I was not sad because I knew that one day I would leave India and see the world. I also knew that by leaving India I would be able to help my family and my country in ways I never could if I remained in India.

Returning home meant returning to my hectic life of chores and school, but once again I sought refuge in my cashew tree with my little transistor radio. After living in comfort in Yemen, however, returning to our small home with no electricity or running water was an adjustment. And while we didn't have sandstorms, we did have powerful monsoons, but I loved those because we would sit on our veranda and watch the wind whipping the towering coconut trees so fiercely that the towering trees swayed like hypnotic dancers. The sky would turn a deep, dark blue or an ominous purplish gray that was occasionally shattered by lightning. And the rains, oh, the heavy rains that drove people home from the fields, hiding their heads in their woven baskets turned upside down to serve as makeshift umbrellas as they hurried for shelter. The poor birds struggled to fly against these powerful winds, while all other wildlife had already gone into hiding. It was as if an angry universe had awoken. And I loved every moment of it.

It was a rather idyllic childhood in many ways, yet my memory of it is one of great stress and puzzlement as I sought to reconcile our life of poverty, hard work, and Christian devotion with the knowledge that I possessed a gifted mind and bore a destiny I did not yet know. I felt as if I was watching my life in the same way I watched the monsoons, and while my future was not yet clear to me, I knew that brighter days were awaiting me, and I was desperately anxious to welcome them.

High school was another turning point in my life, made all the more significant given my young age. I was only around ten when I completed primary school and entered high school, but I had already developed a precocious nature that facilitated many adventures. I was entering St. Augustine's High School, which was fortuitously owned by my grandfather. He had purchased the land and built the school, including about thirty rooms and a large soccer field and other sports facilities.

The school was for grades fifth through twelfth, and for the first time I would go to classes one grade at a time, rather than take lessons from multiple grades simultaneously. My uncle Augustine was the head-master, as he had a master's degree in education, my uncle Christopher was the administrator, and my aunt Stella, Augustine's wife, was the headmistress. It was a most fortunate opportunity for me, as I was able to just walk into my uncle Augustine's office anytime I wanted, which gave me a great deal of stature at the school.

I did very well in school and was particularly good at English, far ahead of the other students. My aunt Stella taught the English class, and she was quite proud of me. She would often ask me to stand up and teach the class because I was so good with the language. I was also quite good at math and whizzed through history and social studies. I barely had to study for exams and always ended up first in my class, year after year, often setting records that have still not been surpassed, at least as far as I know. I got so accustomed to being first in class that it never occurred to me I wouldn't be. To ensure I stayed at the top, I developed a strategy. I would evaluate my classmates to determine who would be number two. Then I would watch that person very closely and find ways to get far ahead of him. I didn't care about the rest of the class—I only cared about that one person who would come in second.

But one year there was a new kid who had joined the school in the middle of the year because his father was the railway train master and had been transferred from another railway station. He wasn't a remarkable kid in any respect and wasn't very social, so I didn't pay him much attention. The year was half-over, and I was focusing on a bright boy I'd been watching all year and was determined to beat. By the time we had our exams, I was so confident I'd beat him that I thought it would be a breeze to come in first yet again.

When the scores were posted, however, I was stunned to see that I had come in second. The new boy whom I hadn't paid any attention to had come in first. I didn't realize how good he was, but there was no denying the fact that he was much smarter than I had assumed. I was mad as hell and had no experience with losing to someone better than me before. I had no idea how to handle it.

I returned home that weekend utterly humiliated. We had a family ritual we performed every quarter, where my mother would fill our largest cup with milk and I, the victor, would drink it down while my brother and sister drank from the smaller cups, and my family congratulated me for my success. But this time, I knew I would not be drinking from the big cup, for I had not been the top student in my class. To add to my anger and humiliation, that very year my sister, Gladis, came home with her scores—and for the first time, she had come in first in her class!

I was furious. I had to watch as Gladis presented the big cup to my mother, who poured some milk into it. George, of course, was never anywhere close to coming in first, so he was used to drinking from the smaller cup. But I was not, so when my mother began to pour some milk into a smaller cup for me, I said, "I'm not going to drink any milk. I don't like milk."

"But, Lenny," my mother said, a barely perceptible smile on her face, "you know you love milk."

"No!" I shook my head defiantly. "I have a stomach upset."

For years my mother would tell that story, laughing as she did so. "This is how bad you were. You just could not take losing even one time." Then she would laugh some more.

I can laugh about it now as well, but at the time all I could think of was how mad I was at my sister because she was first that quarter, and I was not. To this day, whenever I see a glass of milk, that story comes to mind. But as with any failure, the experience taught me well. I learned that when competing for a goal, it is important to not be so quick to judge somebody as inconsequential. People can surprise you. And I learned not to take success for granted, because you can come in first one day but end up second the next. There was one more lesson I learned from my defeat. I made up my mind I would work even harder, and I became all the more determined to be a winner.

High school was an exciting time, and it also gave me my first taste of business. I was a shy young boy, and I did not want to stay shy. I had a great deal of confidence, but in social settings I was hesitant, perhaps because of my young age. My whole driving force was to conquer my limitations, so that I could become the person I was meant to be, the person my grandfather knew I would be from the day I was born.

Thus, when the opportunity presented itself for me to break through my self-imposed social restraints, I seized it.

Once a year our school held an event where they put on a great big feast. Three students were selected every year to be in charge of buying the food and hiring the chef and servers. They even managed the money, for the students paid them directly, and it was up to those in charge to use that money wisely.

Because there was no reward for the hard work of organizing the event, there was no incentive to keep the costs down. The result was that a great deal of money was wasted, and the quality of the food suffered as well.

I realized right away that the students in charge essentially ran the show. Because it was such a time-consuming responsibility on top of all our studies, most students were not interested in all that extra work. But I saw it as an opportunity, so in my last year, I volunteered to manage the food for the event, under the condition that I be able to do it all myself. I promised that I would provide the best food and put on the best event ever. But I would also keep the profit. I didn't want anyone else making decisions, as I already had a plan and wanted complete control over it.

Because I came from a fishing community, I knew a lot of fishmongers and had been well trained by my mother in the art of negotiation for the best fish at the best price. I could also get rice cheap, since so much of it grew near my village.

Now, keep in mind that I was only about thirteen years old at the time, but I was a clever boy. All agreed to my demand, and as promised, we had the best event ever. Best of all, I kept the profit. With that small venture, the capitalist in me had seen the light. I realized that I could earn money as a businessman—I hadn't yet learned the word "entrepreneur"—and that if I provided something people wanted, they could provide me with something I wanted: capital.

I thrived in that school but couldn't wait to get to the big city and get serious about my future. Like any young boy, I wrestled with where

I was going in life and what I would become. I considered becoming a lawyer or going into business and getting an MBA, but I was restless to leave India and make my way in the world. A law degree from India would not be transferable to another country, and an MBA would be limited, as well. I needed a degree that could take me anywhere in the world. That's when it occurred to me that if there's one thing that doesn't change no matter what country it is in, it's the human body. And unlike the textbooks in business or law, which were written in Hindi or Malayalam, all the anatomy and physiology books, indeed, all the medical books, were in English. If I could study medicine in English, I could go anywhere.

Becoming a doctor felt like a natural fit for me. Ever since I was a child, I had loved dressing up as a doctor and being called a doctor. And as I'd grown and become devoted to my faith, healing was something that came naturally to me. I so wanted to help the people in my village, and whenever anyone was sick, they knew they could call on me to take them to the medical college hospital, walk them through the line, and get them to the right person who could help them. While those gestures may have arisen from my Christian faith and my mother's example as someone who was always ready to help others, helping people to get the care they needed had planted in me the seeds to my future. I increasingly realized that I had become a vehicle through which people could find proper health care. Healing people seemed to be the perfect match for my professional interests and my deepening devotion to Christianity and faith. And if I could make money at it, all the better—just as long as I put God's will first and foremost.

CHAPTER 4

Forging My Own Path

In 1965, at the age of fourteen, after finishing tenth grade, I left home. I was awarded the National Merit Scholarship, and my national scores were very high. I was accepted to premed and then to medical college in Trivandrum, the capital city of Kerala. This was permitted under the Indian system.

As excited as I was to begin my medical studies, the thought of being on my own, far from my family, was difficult. I had grown closer to my father in recent years and was still close to my mother and grandfather. I felt like a mature adult intellectually, but emotionally I was still a child, and those two conflicting emotions swirled inside me, but I kept my head high and focused on my future.

My father tried to persuade me to stay, suggesting that I could use the time to study and mature, but I knew it was up to me to fulfill my destiny. I had prayed for the opportunity to see the world and to study medicine, and God had answered my prayers. I could not refuse this chance, no matter how scared I might be.

We packed two bags, and after I hugged my mother and siblings goodbye, my father and I walked barefoot across the paddy fields to the distant bus stop. We waited for the bus, chatting as if we were on our way to the market, but we both knew that this was a momentous ride—I would return for visits, but my home would now be elsewhere, and adulthood awaited me on the other end of that bus ride.

My brother, George, had also been admitted to college, but our family had the money to pay a portion of the room and board for only one of us. Gladis was already in college, studying for a degree in zoology. I had a full scholarship for tuition and two additional scholarships, but I would still need the help of my parents for some of the room and board. Normally, it would be the eldest son who would live on campus, but George had long before stopped picking on me and he loved me dearly, so when my parents suggested that George would live on campus, he said, "No, let Lenny stay there. I will do the daily bus ride."

It was a long ride from our village to Trivandrum, at least an hour and often two hours, which meant arriving late to class and returning home so tired you could barely walk another mile to catch another bus and then make the long trek home. But for the next few years, George willingly endured that long trek back and forth each day so that I could focus on my studies. He recognized and respected my serious pursuit of education. All those years of helping him with his studies had paid off, and I couldn't have loved him more. He had grown from a popular boy who delighted in picking on his little brother to a kind and generous young man who put the needs of others before himself.

Now the time had come for me to make that long trek to what would become my new home. My father and I boarded the bus and rode through the winding, bumpy roads that wove through the villages like a snake in the grass. As we drew closer to the city, the route grew straighter and we rumbled along the long, busier route where businesses and markets increasingly appeared, framed by the sienna-colored earth speckled with the bright green of tall coconut palms and the canopies of shorter cashew trees.

The dust from the road floated like a thick cloud in the unrelenting heat, but it was blazing hot, so we kept all the windows opened. The bus was so packed that our bodies jostled against one another, and people chattered, while the smell of so many hot and sweating people was tempered by the aromatic breads, *dosas*, and ripe mangoes that all of us had packed for later meals.

My mind was not on the bus ride or my physical discomfort, however. My father and I chatted about my plans. I nodded as he reminded me to study hard and stay out of trouble and mind my own business, and I responded with "Yes, Dad...Yes, sir...I will...I know." Yet all I could think of was how excited and nervous and scared I was. But I couldn't let my father know that.

We reached the campus and found the hostel where I'd be living—the Indian version of a dorm—and my father hugged me goodbye, as he was not permitted to stay. I could see in his eyes that he was sad to leave me there all alone, but I also noted the pride in his eyes, and I knew that I would one day make him far more proud. But beneath my own pride, I was so profoundly sad and scared. I watched him from my window, thinking it was the last time I would say goodbye to him as his boy. I was now a man. And I would have to pay my own way from then on.

The room was a simple one, with two thin beds separated by a half wall. Fortunately, it had electricity, and we each had a lamp to study by. Having grown up without electricity, something as simple as an electric lamp was a blessing, and I was thankful for the glow it was to bring me night after night.

I settled down in my room with one other roommate, a very good-looking boy who was much older than me. He had already finished three of five years of college, and he looked upon me much the same as George had looked upon me when we were little. I was just a kid, and I didn't know anything about college or what we had to do or what was going to happen. But I didn't want to be alone, so I talked with him and tried to be friendly and charming, all the while thinking, *Tomorrow when I wake up, I will have to take care of myself.* I was on my own.

Despite the difficulty of those early days in college, I soon settled in and found myself so busy with my studies that I had little time to reflect on all I'd left behind. But I did find time to reflect on all that was up ahead of me, as that was something that drove me to succeed.

My roommate turned out to be from a wealthy family, I learned, and I was envious of his fine clothes and fine shoes. But I didn't let my envy defeat me. Instead, I used it to fuel me into working even harder so that one day I would have such fine clothes and shoes.

I hadn't been there long before I met a priest, Dr. Abraham, who was the warden of the dormitory. He was a very strict warden, but he took a liking to me and I to him, and soon I was working as his assistant of sorts. Whatever help he needed, whether it was putting up a poster in the chapel or making an announcement, I was eager to help. As a result, we grew fairly close, and by spending my time with older people, I began to mature as well.

I also discovered the American Consulate just two miles from the campus. Every month they received new issues of two magazines—*Reader's Digest* and *Life* magazine. I was fascinated by those magazines. *Life* was filled with glamorous photos of people, places, and ideas from a world I'd only dreamed of: the Kennedys, Martin Luther King, the Space Walk. And movie stars: John Wayne, Peter O'Toole, Frank Sinatra. Places: Chicago, Hawaii, New York City. Every page I turned brought a new and mesmerizing image of a world I so badly wanted to be a part of. I imagined myself on the cover of such a magazine, my own life as remarkable as those I read about.

As big and glossy as *Life* magazine may have been, it was the small, compact *Reader's Digest* that brought a more ordinary American world to me; though in the eyes of a young Indian boy, that ordinary world was extraordinary. It was packed with stories and articles about politics, the war in Vietnam, Christianity, and daily life.

I loved the jokes and vocabulary games and quizzes so much that every month I eagerly awaited the day it would arrive. And when that day came, no matter how busy I was, I'd think, *I can't wait one more day!* Setting my studies aside, I would take a bus to the consulate that very day to see the answers to the previous month's quizzes to see if I'd gotten all of them right. And almost always, I had.

I pored over those magazines almost as much as I pored over biology, chemistry, and physics as my brain burned with all the information I was consuming. I had hardly any time for a social life, but I did continue with my faith, praying two or three times a day and going to mass as often as I could. The more I devoted my life to God, I discovered, the easier my life became, so it was not a burden to invest the extra time in my faith. What's more, prayer and faith helped me feel close to my mother, even though we were so far apart.

Fortunately, the food in the cafeteria was fresh and delicious, so as much as I may have missed my mother's cooking, I was not wanting for delicious food. It was even better than the food I'd been able to procure in high school, as the food available in the city was much more varied, the fish was fresh, the meat was delicious, and the vegetables were the best quality.

I so missed my family, and though I did visit every chance I could, my life had taken a turn toward the future, and my childhood was fast receding in the distance as I looked toward medical school and leaving India for good. Then, one morning, my childhood was shattered forever when a knock came on the door to my dormitory. It was a distant family member who had been sent with the news I'd hoped never to hear—my grandfather had passed away and I had to return home.

The news shattered me. Although he was in his late seventies and had lung problems, his death was still a shock. In my mind, my grandfather was immortal, and for him to die before I'd finished medical school was an even greater loss. I had so wanted him to see me graduate, become a doctor, become a rich, successful man—which I was determined to become. Then, suddenly, with a simple knock at the door, that dream was forever silenced. He would never see me graduate, never know the man I was to become. I could barely contain my grief.

There was no time to wait for a bus, so we hired a car and drove straight home. The ride wasn't a long one, just an hour and a half away, but it seemed an eternity as the reality sank in that I would never again sit with my grandfather, never again hear his voice or his wise words, never again see him walk with his gold-plated walking stick, advising the many men and women who sought his counsel.

My family was awaiting my arrival because no decisions could be made until I returned. Moreover, until I returned, his soul could not depart. While I was not the eldest male, and my uncles Augustine and Christopher were his sons, the family knew that I was my grandfather's favorite and intended to take his place of honor in the family. I was still not yet eighteen, but already I felt as if I alone would bear the responsibility for my family's future. The grief, the pressure, the shock all swirled inside me as we drove the same route that had taken me from my village to college and now returned me home.

When we finally reached my grandparents' house, the line of mourners was so long that we had to park quite distant from the house and pass through a long walkway to reach the front entry flanked by mourners on either side of us. I was crying all the way up to the house. When we reached the veranda, I saw his sons, my uncles, standing quietly, welcoming me.

My grandfather was laid out in his casket, resting in the living room. He had been dressed in his finest clothes, covered with a cloth of linen, and his face was pure in its tranquility and wisdom. I immediately fell upon him and held him and cried for the beloved grandfather I would never again see. Eventually, I let go and stepped away, and the casket was carried to the open-air veranda for all the mourners to see. It was then that we began to make plans for his burial, but it was such a difficult moment that I could barely concentrate. All I could think of was how much I wanted him to sit up, to be alive once more, to erase this horrible moment.

For the rest of the day he lay in state on the veranda, as close relatives sat with him to guard his soul. When all the visitations were over, we continued to sit with him until the next day, when he would be buried. As we sat with him, others prepared the walkway where his casket would pass. A canopy of thatch made from the leaves of coconut trees was draped along the lanes that passed through the labyrinth of houses so that if it rained we would not slip on mud while carrying the heavy casket and so that the casket would not be soiled with rain. The church was nearly a mile away, so it was a long procession, but to honor my grandfather, nothing was spared.

The grand, wooden gate leading to my grandfather's house was similarly prepared, covered with coconut leaves to create a beautiful arbor through which people passed. The courtyard and all the rooms of the house were finely decorated as if for a grand festival. My grandfather's body was blanketed in sweet-smelling flowers, but it was a heartbreaking sight I could barely believe I was gazing upon.

We sang hymns and recited prayers, and then, sadly, he was covered with salt from the neck down, and the cover of his coffin was laid across the casket and nailed shut. Then I and the other males of the family carried him along the long walk to the church for the final service. From there, we carried him to his final resting place, where he was set into the ground, and each of us tossed dirt and flowers into his grave.

I had never before suffered such pain and could not imagine my future without him. But my future was before me, and with the death of my grandfather, I took on a greater role in my family. Though not the patriarch, I was considered the heir to my grandfather's wisdom, and from that day forward, my family—even my uncles Augustine and Christopher, as well as my own father—turned to me for advice. I had already gained a great deal of knowledge and knew about a range of things, from politics to current events, the human body and mathematics to making money. Though still a teenager, just sixteen, I had grown wise beyond my years, and my family sought me out for counsel even after I'd returned to school.

After my grandfather's death, my mother had inherited some money, and my father made the decision to at long last retire from his job in Yemen and move back home. But having him back year-round made our small house feel even smaller, so with the money he had from retirement and my mother's inheritance, they decided to buy some land near town, where they would have more space and be less isolated. They found a nice piece of land in the city center and decided on a four-bedroom house that would provide plenty of room for everyone.

Once the time came to get started, however, it became clear that my father was in over his head. He knew how to work with people, but his understanding of construction and what it took to oversee a project like this was just not his strong suit. Plus, by late afternoon he was ready to start drinking, which didn't help matters.

George had finished college and was getting ready to leave Kerala, so he was unable to help. But I already knew that I had a knack for solving problems, so I offered to manage the project. It would mean taking the bus back and forth, which was certainly not convenient, but the opportunity to learn about construction and housing was too good to pass up. After all, I had seen how my grandfather had built up his wealth by buying properties he converted into a post office and school. If I could learn about building a house, I reasoned, I could learn about building a business later on.

After persuading my parents that I could handle the project and still keep up with my studies, I got to work. I found an architect who could draw up a plan and sat with him as we considered where to put the veranda, where the kitchen should be located, where we should put the prayer room. What kinds of shutters should we put on the windows? What kind of roof and what kind of ceiling should we have? What colors should we paint the interior and exterior? What types of materials should be used?

I supervised everything, and as I did, I learned a great deal about how to keep costs down, how to work with permits, what would and would not work and why. I was also supervising adults—an experience that forced me to be less cocky and more mature. I had to not only display confidence, but I had to *be* confident.

Once the building phase began, a new problem emerged. The wood, the bricks, the windows—all the valuable building materials— often had to be left out all night, where anyone could come along and steal them. There was only one solution—on the nights when materials arrived or were stacked up, I would have to sleep there, right out in the open, snakes and all. I didn't like that idea, but my good friend Oswald volunteered to join me those nights, so that's what we did—we camped outside the house, under a jackfruit tree.

I had arranged my classes so I could get off early, and each morning I'd wake around 5:00 a.m., then take the bus back to school an hour away, sit in my classes or take my exams, then jump back on the bus and be back by 3:00 or 4:00 p.m. to manage and pay the workers. At dusk, Oswald would arrive to keep me company, and we'd sleep right there on the ground in the sweltering Indian heat with nothing but a few pillows and light blankets.

My parents paid me for my work, which gave me some spending money, though I never had as much as many of the kids at school. I still couldn't afford to drive a fancy car or wear fine clothes, but I could afford to go to cafés and put some away for future investments. Most importantly, though, I was so proud when the house was finished. I had helped my parents build their dream home! It was so beautiful, with yellow walls and pink trim, large windows and a flat roof. It had been built on a foundation of cement, so there was no dirt floor, and it had a huge well right by the house, so my mother could get water easily without having to haul it from far away.

We christened the house Bethany, a name my parents and I chose from the Bible. Bethany was the town where Martha, Mary, and Lazarus lived—three very different types of people who were united in their love for their fellow villagers and Jesus. That was how I felt our home was—a place that was inclusive of everyone, where people from different faiths and backgrounds and economic classes could come and feel welcome.

My parents were so proud of me, and the joy they felt in making Bethany their home was and remains one of the proudest achievements of my life. When the work was over and my parents moved in, I was finally eligible to begin my clinical medical studies. The only problem was, I wasn't old enough.

Unfortunately, a new law had been passed that required everyone entering clinical medical school to be at least seventeen. I was not yet seventeen, so I had no choice but to wait another year, but I was determined not to waste that year. I focused on advanced physics, chemistry, and biology, confident that doing so would facilitate my understanding of the clinical work ahead of me. It was right around this time that another big job came my way, a group project, and one I was happy to take on. It was up to the men in the family to find a groom for my sister.

It might seem odd to an American, and even to many modern Indians, that a woman does not choose her own husband. Even though we were Christian, it was the Indian custom that families arrange the marriages of their daughters, at least in most cases. Girls don't just go out and date. The reasoning for such an arrangement is that young hearts are not always wise hearts, while a mature parent's judgment usually leads to a better match. As well, marriages in India are as much about the family's status and future as they are about the bride and groom's. In a matrilineal society, who the females marry matters to the family lineage. Thus, the family makes the match.

George was much too busy trying to find a job to be involved in many of the details, but my parents and I set out to find someone who would make a suitable life partner for Gladis, someone worthy of her and from a good family, just as my grandparents had done for my parents.

Gladis had no objection, as arranged marriage was the custom, though of course she would have the final say. So we got to work. We put the word out and found a few young men who were possibilities, but they just didn't sound right. We wanted her to marry someone with a prestigious career, and the most prestigious career in India was a doctor.

Doctors were considered the top choice. After that, an engineer or someone in business. The lowest were lawyers. We decided to avoid those. Teachers and college professors are fairly low, as well, at least from economic terms, but they are well looked upon, so many families will be happy with a teacher or a professor. But doctors—they are another class altogether, especially if they start their own hospital. Such a doctor would make a fine husband for Gladis.

I set to work inquiring of everyone in my professional circle and eventually came upon a young man who had just finished medical school. He was good-looking and came from a good family, so my uncle Augustine, my father, George, and I all met with his family. They were impressed with Gladis and agreed she could make a fine wife for their son. But then came the question of the dowry. In India, the family of the bride has to pay the family of the groom a certain amount of money to compensate them for the loss of a male in the family who will be leaving to join the woman's lineage. The more status and economic security the man and his family have, the greater the dowry. And his family wanted an awful lot of money—far more than my family could afford.

His father was a pretty good negotiator, and at times discussions became heated. He was a little bit more aggressive than most people would be, but we tolerated it. At a certain point, however, it was clear that if Gladis was going to be able to marry this well-off young man, my family would have to give up most of what they owned—including Bethany, my parents' dream home, which I had only recently helped them to build. The home had been built on two and a half acres of land, with a lot of property surrounding it. It had a nice gate and many coconut trees and highly fertile land with a lot of produce. Anyone would be proud to live there, and my parents loved their home.

Over the next few days, we pondered the options before us.

"No, we can't do that!" my father insisted, unwilling to relinquish Bethany.

"We cannot. That is our home. And when we pass, our property must be divided equally among all three of you. We cannot give up our home."

I proposed a plan.

"I don't want any of this," I told him. "I really want to give it to her. Because one day I will have my own, and I will be sure the family is taken care of. And we can have them include a stipulation in the document that Mom and Dad can live there as long as they're alive. They cannot be moved, and no one can come live there without their permission. But after they've passed, Bethany will go to my sister and her family."

George remained silent, as he wasn't much of a negotiator or decision maker, and Augustine said nothing as he had no say in the matter. It was up to my mother and father, but they trusted me. They had already seen enough in me to know I was ambitious. They trusted I'd make good on my word and take care of the family. As they considered the matter, they were sufficiently influenced by me that they agreed. If I was willing to forgo my rights to the home and George was as well, then it would be in everyone's best interest to include Bethany in the dowry, as long as they could remain there for the rest of their lives.

At that point, it was simply a matter of persuading George. He was understandably upset at the prospect of losing his share of the inheritance, but we managed him. I assured my parents that I would help him secure a good position in the government. Under the socialist system in India, the oil industry, railway, airline, and postal systems were all owned by the government. All he needed to do was excel on his entrance exams.

"Don't worry," I told my parents. "I will coach him and tell him exactly what to do for the exams, so that he'll get the highest score and get a good job." Added to that, I reminded my father that his own connections in the Middle East could help George as well, since Dubai was growing, and jobs would be flourishing there, a point my father found convincing.

Once my parents were on board, we presented our plan to George and persuaded him that he would fare much better with such a plan and with our sister financially secure in a good marriage.

And so it was that the dowry was secured, and Gladis was married. She had been teaching marine biology and zoology at the university by that time, but she gave up her job and began a happy life with a good man who to this day has been a wonderful husband and father.

In the meantime, I counted the days until I would turn seventeen and start my clinical medical studies. When that day came, I started medical school and spent the next few years buried in medical books and doing clinical rounds. I had finally reached my first major life goal, and that accomplishment gave me the drive to continue on my path.

I hadn't been in medical school long before I took it upon myself to be the medical liaison for the Christian fisherman community in the region, a high-status position that gave me considerable social influence, despite my young age. In India, while everyone receives free medical care, the health programs are so poorly run in some parts of the country that people can wait hours for care, only to be told at 4:00 p.m. that the clinic is closed and they must return the next day—an especially maddening event given that some people typically hike or bus several hours just to reach the clinic.

But as medical liaison, I was able to get people to the head of the line, so soon everybody I knew loved me. If they were sick or injured, all they had to do was get word to me and I would arrange for them to be seen promptly at the clinic. We had no cell phones in those days, so reaching me was not always easy, but somehow people managed to find me every day, keeping me all the more busy.

I thrived in my new career and for the first time felt that I was fulfilling my destiny. I felt as if I had at long last finished a race and reached my goal. But with that victory came another race before me, the race to practice medicine. I absorbed everything, from books to bodies as I learned the healing arts. Seeing patients and tending to their wounds or treating their illnesses brought me great pride to know that I was serving the Lord through my gift of healing, and I knew that the more I used that gift, the more gifts the Lord would return to me. And that gift came, more often than not, in the form of the caring and wonderful people who came into my life.

I did not have much of a social life. I could not commit myself to a girlfriend or to anyone at that point. For one, I was incredibly busy with my studies, and since the food at the medical school was mediocre, I had no choice but to improve it.

Each year, there was a system where one to three students were chosen to run the cafeteria and were responsible for the menu, procurement of food items, and the finances.

I knew I could do this job, partly based on my high school experience running an event and providing a good meal for a low cost. I volunteered for the position and took over the responsibility of running the cafeteria.

So I met with some fishmongers I knew, as well as farmers, and negotiated for the best food I could find. I also hired the best cooks I could find, and I was able to do it all for a low price. The food was so fresh and tasty that I soon became the golden boy, and my popularity soared, along with my social confidence. I also made a lot of money, because due to my connections with the fishmongers and rice sellers and my clever negotiations, I could keep the prices low all year long.

I was so busy there wasn't much time left in the day, but I was making enough money to help pay for my room and board. I had made such a good profit, in fact, that I was able to buy a Java, which was a Czechoslovakian motorbike. It was the finest motorbike I'd ever seen— sleek and lightweight but fast and beautiful. "Man's best friend" was how the bike was advertised, and like my transistor radio had been, my motorbike quickly became my new best friend. I painted the whole thing bright green so that everyone would know it was my bike when they saw it, and I rode it everywhere. There were no traffic rules. There weren't even any traffic lights. Instead, the roads were filled with buses and rickshaws and cows and horses and bicycles all going every which way, so getting anywhere was a headache. It was just anarchy. But on my little green Java, I could whip through any roadblock, go anywhere I wanted, and best of all, I no longer had to take the bus or train back home. I could just hop on my bike and drive myself there. That was the end of my shyness, as I became quite popular because everyone wanted a ride on my bike. It was only built for two, but I always had three or four people on it. I managed to squeeze them on, all of us standing, and we went everywhere on that bike.

As busy as I was with my studies and social life, however, I was restless. I wanted to leave India. I didn't fit in there. When I looked around at all the people I'd gone to school with, I could see that they were stuck in small jobs, doing well enough, but no one was excelling. I wanted to excel. And I couldn't do that in India. I wanted to go to England, where I could study medicine with even greater minds.

There was one other idea driving me, one that dominated all other thoughts—I still wanted to know what it was about the British that enabled them to dominate my nation. We so outnumbered them, yet they had conquered us. As much as I was fascinated with America, the whole idea of the British having conquered us took control of my thoughts. *Who are these British people?* I wondered. I could not shake the sense that I had to go to London to better understand what it was about the British that had made such a small group so powerful.

I knew that if I went to England, it would be up to me to fit in. My fascination with the British included a deep desire to be like them—to no longer feel conquered and dominated, but to feel, instead, empowered. If I was going to fit in with them, I thought, I should learn British culture. I already knew how to play soccer, but the wealthy British all played tennis. So I decided that while I was busy learning medicine and running the cafeteria, I'd learn to play tennis as well.

I found a tennis club not too far away, one that required riding my motorbike through the city. So when my studies were done, I'd grab my tennis racket, fasten it to the side of my motorbike, and zip in and out of the traffic like some kind of crazed daredevil. The traffic in India, as I've said, is absolutely chaotic, and with no rules or lights, just passing through an intersection is a gamble with death, but somehow I always made it to the tennis courts and back without a scratch. I became convinced that if I survived those roads, I would live to be a very old man. More to the point, the more I rode that motorbike, the more I came to realize that, over and over again, God was sparing my life, which meant there was a purpose I had to fulfill. I came to see that God had chosen me for something, whether that be healing or something else, but one thing was certain. God was on my side.

God was also on the side of my Jewish friends, who were increasingly being persecuted by a group of local Muslims and Hindus who wanted to drive them out. There are large populations of Hindus, Muslims, Christians, Buddhists, Sikhs, and those who practice Jainism, and for the most part, we all got along very well and there was a great deal of religious tolerance in India. But this one particular group was an exception, and their persecution of the Jews could not go unaddressed.

As a minority Christian, I empathized with the Jews, and from the time I was a child, I had always had friends from all faiths. And I certainly had no ill feelings about Jews. After all, Jesus was a Jew, so to treat them badly was to denounce Jesus. So when the Muslims made threats against the local synagogue, I knew I had to do something.

Now, you must understand the history of the Malabar Jews in Kerala. They are also known as the Cochin Jews because most of them lived in the city of Cochin, a busy center of finance and trade, where they had settled centuries ago, after fleeing attacks from the Muslims who wanted to take over the pepper trade. So while we lived together peacefully, there was an underlying tension between the Jews and the Muslims that had been ongoing for ages.

The Muslims had been in southern India since the seventh century, and the Cochin Jews had been in the country since the time of King Solomon, coming to India a thousand years before Christ. They were the oldest group of Jews in all of India. They still worshipped in the synagogues that were built in the thirteenth and sixteenth centuries—and it was one of these synagogues that had come under threat.

Now, as I've noted over the years, I had become quite close to the fishermen in my community. Not only had my mother taught me well about how to bargain for the lowest price for the freshest fish and I'd been trading with them regularly while running the cafeteria, but now that I was the medical liaison for the fisherman community, I was the one who got health care for the fishermen. In short, I looked out for them, and they looked out for me.

It was a good thing to have the fishermen on my side because men who set sail on the ocean in small boats to capture fish of all sizes are not ordinary men. They are tough, strong, and have a code all their own—if you cross them, one might hack you to death with a machete and toss you into the waves as bait for the day's catch, at least that is the reputation these rugged men have.

When I learned of the threats against the synagogue, I saw it as a threat against my friends and my history, and I knew what God wanted of me. So I met with the fishermen, who are all Christian, and asked if they could provide protection for the synagogue. Without hesitation, they assured me they would be sure no harm came to the Jews.

We went together to the synagogue and mapped out the area to assess how much manpower we'd need. Once we knew the area, our plan was set. For the next several nights, when the sun began to set around 8:00 p.m., the fishermen arrived en masse and blocked off a three-block area. The message was clear—these people are protected, the synagogue is protected, and anyone who dares harm them will face the fishermen.

In less than a week, the threats came to an end. I felt I had done God's work. Viewing religion as the vehicle through which we each reach God, I felt I had done my part in bringing us together. As devout a Christian as I am, I have never felt a person's religion made them any less holy than anyone else. I liken it to making phone calls using a smartphone. One may have a different carrier than someone else, yet we are all using our devices to try to reach God. We all, in our faith, know that our connection will never be severed. For me, Christianity is the vehicle, or cellular connection, I use to reach God. It is the only faith I know, the faith I was born into and raised in. But ultimately we are all in it together in our collective faith in God. Thus it was through the help of the fishermen that I did my part in reminding some that the Jews would be left in peace to worship God, just as any Christian or Muslim would expect to be left to pray in peace.

My many years in medical school kept me so busy that even now, half a century later, I cannot clearly recall my studies as much as the transformative nature that period had on me as I went from teenager to young adult, gaining experience in business and settling disputes, just as my grandfather had done before me. I felt as if his spirit had entered my soul and he guided me toward my future.

After graduating from medical school, I worked for the next two years in a private hospital as an assistant doctor. I stayed busy through my work and continued to help my family, but my restlessness was great. As my residency drew to a close, the future I had spent my life awaiting was upon me. It was time to leave India and start that life—in London, England.

PART II

SENT FROM GOD

"...So we can only pray, if we are Hindus, not that a Christian should become a Hindu, but our innermost prayer should be that a Hindu should become a better Hindu, a Muslim a better Muslim, and a Christian a better Christian."

Mahatma Gandhi

❧ CHAPTER 5 ❧

An Unexpected Friend

I had no real plan. My family didn't have the money to send me to London, and I sure didn't have it. It was a difficult situation. In the past, I always had a plan; I could always figure a way to solve a problem. But this time I was stumped because I didn't know anyone who could help me.

By this point, my uncle Augustine was the family patriarch, and he felt I should be married. He and my parents began looking for a wife for me, and while they did arrange for me to meet a couple of girls with considerable dowries and impressive wealth—girls who came from families who owned big factories and businesses—it just didn't feel right. Just as I wasn't going to marry someone for a dowry, I also felt deep in my heart that my path was not in India. I had to remain focused on my medical education and launch my career before I contemplated marriage. But in the meantime, I went through the motions of courtship with various women my family had chosen to satisfy them that I would indeed get married. We just disagreed on when that marriage would be.

With no foreseeable solution, I turned to God. I prayed to God to show me a way. I implored God to help me reach the United Kingdom, somehow, some way. But the more I thought about it and the more I prayed and the more my family pressured me to marry, the more hopeless my situation felt. But hopeless or not, I maintained my faith in God. I knew that if I kept my faith, a way would be shown to me.

Then one day I found myself hanging out with an acquaintance of mine, a friendly guy named Frederick, though we called him Freddy. I didn't know Freddy well, but well enough to take a seat with him and chat for a bit.

We were chatting about school or some such thing, when Freddy said something, and I realized I hadn't been paying any attention to our conversation. That's when he asked me, "What's wrong, Lenny? Why are you so thoughtful? You're not really here. Your mind is somewhere else."

He was right. My mind was somewhere else, and I decided to share my worries with him. "I'm sorry, Freddy. You're right, my mind is somewhere else. The problem is, I really want to go to the United Kingdom," I told him. "I want to practice medicine in London, but I don't know how to make that happen. I'm trying to find a way, and I know it will come to me, but I just have to continue to meditate and connect with my soul and the universe to find a way."

Freddy's face brightened. "That's interesting," he said. "You know, my father works in London."

I raised my brows. "I didn't know that."

"Yes, he works for the British Rail. He's a ticket collector, and I can call him. I think he'll help you."

"Really? You'd do that?" I asked him. "Do you really think he could help me?"

Freddy assured me he'd see what he could do, and my hopes soared. How a ticket collector for the railway could possibly help me, I had no idea, but it was the first connection I had to London, and my spirits soared. I prayed harder than ever that evening and the next few days after that, imploring the Lord to open the heart of this ticket collector in London I didn't even know so that he might help me.

A few days later, Freddy came by. "I've got good news," he said, and from the smile on his face, I knew it to be true. Before I could even respond, he said, "My dad says he'd like to sponsor you when you come to London."

I was stunned. I needed a sponsor to get there, but this man did not even know me!

"Really? Oh, Freddy, that's wonderful! Your father is such a good man," I replied. But then my smile softened, as my problems weren't entirely resolved. "But I'm not ready to go yet. I don't even have a place to live. I'm going to have to find something first."

"That's not a problem," he replied. "He said you can stay at his place, and he'll do whatever is needed to help you get settled."

I was shocked. I had expected the Lord to answer my prayers, but not this easily, not this quickly, not this wondrously! I hardly even knew Freddy, yet his father was offering me a home and sponsorship in the United Kingdom. I was overjoyed.

I also had to get moving. I realized that I couldn't wait too long if I were to accept the offer, so I had to get ready for the big move. The first thing I would have to do was buy a ticket, and that would cost me about $2,000, which was more money than I'd ever seen. Fortunately, I knew one way to come up with half that. I would have to sell my motorbike. I hated to part with it, but I couldn't afford to take it with me, so selling it was the only option. As for the other half, it was time to turn to God and to my family.

I was afraid to ask my parents for the money. It wasn't because I thought they'd be upset. Quite the contrary. I feared they would take unnecessary risks to find the money. They couldn't sell their home, as that had already been bequeathed to Gladis, but I didn't want them to take out a loan or sell anything they might have of value because they had so little.

"Don't worry," I assured my parents instead. "I'm going to leave. I have to. And I'll find the money somehow. God has answered my prayers so far, and he will continue to answer them in his own time and in his own way."

My mother smiled. Since I'd been a small boy, she was determined that I would find the Lord and gain strength through prayer, and her efforts had paid off. And I was confident that not only would she pray for me, as well, but that God would pay special attention to her prayers, because her devotion was near saintly.

It wasn't long before my mother's prayers were also answered. Although I hadn't spoken to him about my dilemma, my uncle Christopher heard of it and he paid me a visit.

"I'll loan you the money, Lenny," he told me. "But you must pay me back. And I trust that you will because you are an honorable man."

His generosity was my saving grace. I assured my uncle that he would see every rupee back and then some, and once I sold my bike, I had the money that I needed to get to London. I would have nothing when I got there, but I figured if I just bought the ticket, I would deal with the rest once I got there. At least I'd be in England, and I had a place to stay. I would take the medical exam so that I could practice in England, and somehow, some way, I knew I would survive.

During this time, I was driven and focused on a single goal—getting to England and practicing medicine in the British system. I was determined to not just be a doctor there, but to be a great doctor, someone of high regard. To do that, I would need to work hard, pray hard, and trust in the Lord to guide me toward my destiny.

I couldn't wait to get on that plane. Since I would have no money, I knew I would have to take the medical exams to qualify to practice in the British system as soon as possible. But one thing stumped me— understanding British accents! I was fluent in English and had been for most of my life, but I had been taught English by Indians, and the English I spoke and heard was almost always with an Indian accent. Once I started working in England, I would have to understand the other doctors and the nurses, not to mention the patients, but I strained to make sense of what they were saying.

But I had always approached problems as something to be solved, so I got tapes and spent the next several weeks listening and listening and listening to as much British English as I could until it began to sound natural to me. As it did, my confidence returned. I knew I would be fine. But how I would make it until then, I wasn't sure, since I had no money.

Then, just a few days before it was time to leave, I received a large envelope from my sponsor, Mr. Joseph, Freddy's father, with whom I'd been in correspondence. Inside the envelope were instructions on where Mr. Joseph would be when I got to London, with a map and a picture of him so I would recognize him. Among all these papers was one more thing—one hundred British pounds in cash to spend on the journey there!

I was stunned. And so touched. This man was an angel. I do not say that figuratively, for he had come into my life so miraculously and been so generous and kind to me, a total stranger, that there is no other explanation than Mr. Joseph had been sent by God to guide me on my path. I cried in joy at the kindness of this new friend who was making my future possible.

The day came to say goodbye to my family. Parting from my family, especially my mother and father, was like the day I'd watched my father walk away after he'd left me at the hostel in Trivandrum all those years before. Many years had passed. I had gained and lost so much—I had gained an education, experience as an entrepreneur, and even experience in construction, helping my parents to build their dream home. But I had lost my innocence, my childhood, and most of all, my grandfather, a loss that would haunt me all my life.

I felt as if I was already a wizened elder myself, when in fact I was still just starting my life and career. My, how I would miss my family. I would so miss those trips to St. Augustine's Shrine with my mother. I would miss her wonderful *doshas* and fish stews. I would miss her gentle face.

We cried and hugged and said our goodbyes, but we all knew that we were not parting for good. I was a penniless young doctor, but I knew beyond a doubt that I was on my way to a future that would change all our lives.

It was my first flight. Just as I had sailed across the Arabian Sea as a child, my face pressed against the glass as I took in the infinite waters that enveloped me, now I pressed my face against the glass of the jet and fathomed the infinite skies that cradled me to my destiny as if God himself were piloting the plane to heaven.

But getting to this heaven of mine took two stops, and the food was, at best, palatable, not heavenly. I didn't mind though. I was finally on my way.

When I landed at Heathrow Airport, I was shocked by the cold. I had never known such cold, and I owned no warm clothes, as there was no need for them in India. I had no idea how I'd manage to stay warm. I passed through the crowds, finding my way just as Mr. Joseph had instructed me. He had told me to meet him at the baggage claim, so I followed the signs, all in English, which I could easily read. Already I felt I belonged. Except, of course, for the cold.

Then I saw him. I recognized him from his photo, a fairly short man, with a big round belly that suited his warm smile. He immediately struck me as a friendly, personable person, which, of course, I knew already from the kindness and generosity he had extended to me.

He was holding a big blanket, and the moment I approached him, he wrapped the blanket around me.

"Here," he said. "I thought you might need this for the cold."

I couldn't believe his thoughtfulness. It was as if he had read my mind. He truly was an angel.

After a few pleasant words of greeting, he said, "Come, let's get on the train and we go!" He picked up my bag and escorted me to the British Rail, explaining that he lived in East London, where the immigrants and poor people live.

"We're in West London right now," he said, "where the prosperous people live. Ahh, well, one day, young man, you will live in West London, as well. But for now, we must cross the city!"

He was so jovial and generous with his heart and home that I felt as if I were indeed already prosperous, to be invited to stay with him in his East London home. Yet the whole train ride there was but a blur because all I could think of was the amazing fact that I was finally in London. I was really, truly there!

We reached our stop and got off and walked a few blocks until we came to an old brick building. We went inside and walked up the dark steps until we reached his apartment, where he had explained that he lived with four other men, each with his own room. He unlocked his room, which had one bed and a hot plate on the floor.

"You will sleep here, on the bed," he told me, "and I will sleep on the floor."

"No, Mr. Joseph, I cannot," I began to protest, but he cut me short.

"I insist. You are my guest, and my guests do not sleep on the floor."

I nodded, knowing better than to argue. I was so honored and humbled.

"There is a bathroom downstairs, and we all share it. I cook here, and eat here, but there is a common room if you want some company, and you may eat there if you'd like."

I stared at this wretched, wonderful place. Their poverty was so great, the amenities so bare, and yet the generosity of his spirit was profound. I was truly in the presence of a Christ-like spirit—someone who had little yet gave so much, putting himself last so that his guest, a stranger, might be comforted.

That night he made a pot of rice on the hot plate, and when it was done, he set it aside and made a simple but tasty chicken dish that we ate with the rice on the floor as if it were a feast. I was so hungry, and so touched, that I devoured it with relish. I had before, and have since, eaten spectacular, lavish meals, and yet I remember few of them as clearly as I do this simple rice and chicken dish enjoyed on the floor of an East Indian tenement with a railway worker I barely knew. When I fell asleep in his bed that night, I thanked God for sending this kind man to me, as he softly snored on the floor beside me.

✔ CHAPTER 6 ✖

In the Company of Royals

The next day, it was back to reality. I had no time to take in the sights of London or play the tourist. For that matter, I had no time to even be jet-lagged. I had to find out where the exam for admission to practice in England would be, as I had to pass that exam in order to find a job.

Before he left for his work with the railway, Mr. Joseph gave me some tips on where to catch the bus and where to go to inquire about the exam, and then he left me to my own devices. I was relieved to know that he would not expect me to spend a lot of time with him, as I had to focus on my studies and he understood that. He was not looking for a companion but truly wanted to be of help, which was exactly what I needed.

After a confusing but exciting day of running here and there, I learned that in two weeks from that day, there was an exam in Edinburgh, Scotland. There was no exam coming up in England, as they rotated the exam from England to Scotland to Wales to Northern Ireland. "Okay," I told myself, "I will start preparing, and in two weeks I will go to Scotland."

Of course, I had no idea how I would get to Scotland, and I could ill afford the trip, as the hundred pounds Mr. Joseph had given me was disappearing faster than I'd anticipated, just with the cost of telephone calls, bus fare, and a bite to eat here and there. Fast running out of money, I did what I always do when faced with such a dilemma. I prayed.

And as always, my prayers were answered. "No problem," Mr. Joseph said over dinner when I told him what I'd discovered that day. "I work for British Rail. I will get you a free ticket on the Flying Scotsman."

The Flying Scotsman, he explained, was the fastest train from London to Edinburgh, arriving in only four hours. "You will love it!" he assured me. "You will be flying, just flying, all the way to Scotland on that train!" His joy was as great as if he himself would be on that speeding train. I couldn't wait.

I spent the next two weeks just walking around, getting to know the city. I struck up a conversation with anyone I could just so I could understand the accent better. But sometimes it was really difficult to understand, especially when someone spoke with a cockney accent. I was fluent in English, but that accent sounded like another language altogether.

I especially asked about health and medicine, so I had a better sense of the health system and how people understood illness and disorders. Shifting from the medical system in India to the medical system in England was a bigger leap than I'd imagined, but my training had been in Western medicine, so it wasn't so much thinking about the body and healing differently as much as getting to know the NHS, the National Health System.

In India, health care is much more disorganized and dependent upon where a person lives, what kind of access they have to safe drinking water and food, and how much money they have, whereas in the U.K., everyone has access to safe food and water and the right to see a general practitioner. Sure, lots of people I spoke with complained about their doctors, but more often than not they were happy to explain to me the virtues of their health system and how it worked. The conversations were like a crash course in both English and the NHS.

In the meantime, I didn't see much of Mr. Joseph. He left for work early every morning and worked twelve-hour days. We had a good relationship, though, but between our schedules, we didn't cross paths often except to sleep at night. But he did put me in touch with some White people he knew who owned shops and businesses, and that enabled me to spend time with them, practice my English, and get to talk to all the people who came and went in their shops.

The two weeks passed quickly, and the time came to go to Edinburgh. Mr. Joseph had been correct; the train went so fast it practically flew. About all I could see out the window was a streak of countryside as it whizzed right past me.

The test was a tough one, and though tests were something I knew I was good at, most people have to take the test three or four times, so as I waited for the results, I did worry a bit. I couldn't afford not to pass, as I had no money and needed to start work. A few days later, on a Monday morning, the test results came in.

I'd passed! I was thrilled! I'd passed on the first try and could start work right away as a medical resident in London, the first stage in a doctor's career. Though I'd already had a residency in India, in order to practice in England, I would have to have another residency. Given the vast difference in the technology, however, I was fine with that, as I knew there was still a lot to learn.

As my life's path accelerated and so much good fortune was coming my way, I was also coming face-to-face with the dark side of my journey. As a Christian, I had grown up as a minority in India, one from a poor family despite my grandfather's stature. Through my grandfather I had become accustomed to high status and the comforts of finer living, but my parents were not well off, and with my father in Yemen for so many years, the poverty that my mother struggled with had left its mark on me. I had a horrid fear of poverty and a sense that my place in the world was among the most successful. Yet as a minority in my home country, there was always this gnawing sense of not fitting in. I loved and embraced people of all faiths and classes, yet I cannot deny that I envied those from wealthier families—indeed, that envy helped propel me forward. It fueled my determination to succeed.

Yet once in England, as much as I was so proud of having finally made it to London, and of passing such a difficult medical exam, I couldn't help but become aware of the fact that immigrants were second-rate, and I was unmistakably an immigrant. Immigrants did not work in the best hospitals in London. Immigrants did not even work in the East End. Immigrant doctors were invariably forced to accept positions on the outskirts of town, in the distant suburbs and small towns like New Castle and Bedford, where the wealthy were unlikely to have to be treated by a dark-skinned doctor speaking with an accent. That was the path I was expected to pursue. And that was the path I was determined not to take. I wanted to work in London. I had come this far. I was not about to bow my head and go away.

I made up my mind to have the courage to present myself to everyone and anyone who might have a residency position available. I sent out applications to every hospital in London, working from sunrise to sunset and late into the night, leaving no respectable position overlooked. It was a numbers game, I reasoned, and if I was rejected by 99 percent of the places I applied to, it meant I would be accepted by 1 percent, and I only needed one job, one good job. As good fortune would have it, it wasn't long before that one job presented itself.

I was offered a residency position at a hospital in London treating diabetes and hypertension. At that point in my career, I hadn't settled on a specialization, and treating chronic diseases seemed to be a good introduction into Western medicine and the NHS. I would also be working in the emergency room as needed, which is one of the most high-pressured and intense positions in any hospital. I couldn't have been happier. I would receive a great deal of clinical experience, and that was exactly what I was looking for. And on top of it all, the position came with housing—a beautiful two-bedroom apartment.

I'd been in London only three weeks, and already I had passed my exams and found an excellent residency in the city and an apartment. I bade farewell to Mr. Joseph, who I'm sure was happy to have his room back but who couldn't have been more gracious. I assured him I would never forget his kindness—nor did I. He was my friend and mentor, and we kept in touch regularly. He would remain in London for a few more years before returning to India, but I made sure to repay him for his generosity many times over.

The apartment I'd been assigned was a simple but impressive one in an upscale neighborhood in the West End, though in my young eyes at the time, it was the most luxurious home I had ever lived in. There was a nice kitchen with a dishwasher, and there was a washer and dryer, but I had absolutely no idea how to use any of them. I'd never really cooked for myself and had no idea how the dishwasher worked. As for the washing machine and dryer, they might as well have been space rockets, they were so bewildering to me. In any event, I was too busy to concern myself with learning how to work any of those machines. There was a laundry service that picked up our laundry once a week, so all I had to do was leave it outside my door. As for cooking, I had no need to learn that, either, as there was a catering service that delivered meals and there were a dozen restaurants on every block. My interest wasn't in cooking and cleaning. They even had a maid service, so I didn't need to do any housecleaning. I was grateful for those services, as my interest was in healing people and working hard to succeed in my career.

In the meantime, I had another test to take. This one was going to be one of the toughest tests I'd ever taken—the driving test. While I knew how to drive, as I've said, in India there were no rules of the road. We'd just step on the gas and go. But in England, it was another story altogether. Not only did they have stoplights, but they had all sorts of rules about how many feet you had to be from an intersection, from the car in front of you, from the curb, how to park, how to turn, how to signal. It was so confusing. But like every test I took, I studied for it, and fortunately, I did pass, but let's just say no one was offering me a big cup of milk for my victory! I was just relieved to have answered enough questions correctly that they gave me my license. The next step was buying a car, but I would have to wait to save up the money for that.

The next couple of weeks passed in a blizzard of work, which was at once intense, challenging, and wonderful. I learned more in those two weeks than I'd probably learned in my medical career so far. Then, on a Thursday, I received my first paycheck—about five hundred pounds. I had never seen that much money in my life! This was in 1975, and five hundred pounds back then was the equivalent of about 4,200 pounds today—over $5,000! I held the check in my hands and couldn't believe I was reading it correctly, but I knew that it was real. I told my boss, the consulting physician, that I needed to take a one-hour break, and as I'd already been working long hours, he didn't mind.

I cried all the way to the bank. I was literally weeping. I just couldn't wait to send that money to my parents. It was one of the most joyful days of my life to know that I could change my parents' life with that check.

After cashing the check at the bank and keeping 150 pounds for myself, I went straight to the post office and wired the rest to my parents. Oh, how I wish I could have seen their faces when they received that money! That first paycheck marked the beginning of my realization that if I worked hard enough, there would be no limit to how much I could earn and how many people I could help in my life.

I had only just begun my work as a resident, but in just those two short weeks, I saw that there were two pathways for the young doctors like me doing our residency in the hospital. One was to continue as a resident and become a general practitioner or work for the government in a clinic or some other setting. The other was to pursue postgraduate studies, take higher exams, and become a consultant, like the consulting physician who supervised us. There was no question which path I was going to take. I would do my postgraduate studies in England and become a consultant. And while all the consultants were older men in their forties and fifties, I didn't see any reason to wait that long. Now I had a new goal.

In the meantime, I worked hard, and it wasn't long before I had enough money to buy an old used car. It wasn't much to look at and didn't run very well, but it would get me across town, which was all I needed for the time being.

So there I was, in England not more than six weeks, and already restless to go even further. My imagination couldn't be contained—but I also knew that imagination is not enough. I would need to turn that imagination into action.

I continued my residency, absorbing as much knowledge as possible. I was amazed at the technology available in this big, modern hospital—far beyond anything I'd worked with in India. I was also amazed at what the lab panels could determine—in India, if we sent in blood work, it came back with little information. But here, sending in a blood, urine, or tissue sample produced extensive information about the patient's state of health.

I was astounded at the medical advancements and began to realize the role that this technological advancement had in enabling the British Empire to colonize my country—while it wasn't advancements in health care that facilitated their conquering of India, they clearly had technological capabilities in trade, transportation, communication, and military that enabled such a small nation to gain control over one much larger. And I wanted to be on the side of those advances.

There was something else that struck me about England's ability to rule my people—they had a marked cultural advantage. Many people in India believe that when a person is born, his or her destiny is determined by the stars, so there is no point in trying to change it. For those who embrace that belief, they often just go through the motions of life, rather than strive for more.

In contrast, I found the British way more reserved and purposeful. Most educated British people are always strategizing and planning. Their inquisitive nature, particularly about other cultures, may have influenced their eagerness to venture from their homelands to define their own destiny. Of course, I am not dismissing the very real conquest of my country and the British desire to seize its resources. Indian culture has a deep-rooted faith in the concept of mind over matter. I have yet to see someone build an amazing building with mind alone. It takes materials, labor, technology, and money to build anything—and England found both labor and resources in our land. There were many features of British colonialism that I found disturbing. But what had always intrigued me was the cultural psychology of the respective nations that had contributed to that conquest. But for me, colonial occupation was personal. I wanted to live a life that ensured I would never be conquered by anyone. My view reflects another aspect to Indian cultural psychology that has enabled us to build the most lavish palaces and fascinating civilization. We have the capacity for greatness, as our minds are sharp and our vision great. As Ross Perot, the billionaire founder of Electronic Data Systems and Perot Systems who once ran for president, would quip, "Every Indian is born with a computer chip in his brain, and it takes just a dollar sign to activate it."

Though I wanted to value our faith in God and thousands of years of culture and mysticism while still being a modern-day Indian, I also wanted to be someone who plans and strategizes and networks to make the world a more prosperous place than we found it. I knew by living and practicing in England, I could represent the best of both worlds.

Toward that end, my exposure to modern health care continued to grow. I was also gaining expertise in chronic health care and trauma, while building my social network. It became clear that in order to succeed, I would need to work under the supervision of someone exceptional, someone really well connected and famous. That would be the key to opening doors for me, so I made myself known far and wide. I introduced myself to everyone I came into contact with and researched who the most influential physicians were in the city of London. Sure enough, it wasn't long before I met a physician who was well connected with the royal family, a distant cousin in fact, and a knight. His name was Sir Scott Gray, and he proved to be another of the kind souls who guided me toward my destiny.

Sir Gray was a short, balding man with a fringe of graying hair and a round face accented by the kindest smile. He spoke with a distinct, proper British accent that reflected his aristocratic background. Sir Gray controlled three hospitals, and he was quite impressed with me and agreed to supervise me, so I began working for him. We worked on a six-month rotation, so every six months, I was transferred to another unit, which enabled me to gain a wide range of skills. The work was hard, but I worked hard. Sir Gray was a wonderful mentor and an excellent doctor, but he only came in on Tuesdays and Thursdays to check on things. He specialized in internal medicine and cardiology, which meant that many of the patients were quite sick. I made sure he saw the sickest, and after he'd checked on them and I brought him up to date on the patients and staff, he'd sign off on the patients and be gone again. Consequently, I found myself pretty much running things in his absence, supervising a staff of about forty young doctors, even though I was barely beyond my residency. He was so impressed with my work that he appointed me registrar, thus formalizing my supervisory role.

Meanwhile, in my spare time, I studied for the next exam—the Membership of the Royal College of Physicians exam. Passing the MRCP exam qualifies a physician as a member of the Royal College of Physicians—a status that is necessary in order to specialize. More than half the physicians who take the exam fail it, but I had never failed an exam and wasn't about to start with that one. So I studied hard and passed. I then realized that I could take the same exam in Dublin and could have a second MRCP, so I took the MRCP exam there and again passed. I liked Dublin so much I moved there and briefly took a job in a hospital. I wasn't there long, however, before Sir Gray urged me to return, so six months later, I packed up once again and returned to London.

It just so happened that Sir Gray lived in a nice little palace with his wife and children, and every Sunday afternoon he would invite me over to play a game of croquet on his beautiful croquet court. After we'd play, we dined in his great hall with an ever-changing array of wealthy White people who were well connected in British society. These social connections were not only invaluable to me as I progressed in my career, but more importantly, I gained the Western social skills of the upper class, and as I mingled with these British aristocrats, my confidence soared. I no longer felt like a poor young immigrant. I was at ease with some of the wealthiest and noblest gentlemen and -women in all of England, and they were at ease with me, Dr. Peters. I had no need to look up to them.

I was also having a lot of fun. I was making a lot of money and continuing to send money back to my family regularly, but no matter how much I sent, I seemed to make even more. I was so happy and proud of my success, and I wasn't afraid to show it off. I had lived most of my life in envy of the beautiful clothes and fancy cars and fine dining that my Indian classmates had enjoyed, so I wasted no time in buying flashy clothes for myself and dining in the best restaurants. As for my old beat-up car, it broke down more often than it started, so as soon as I'd saved the money, I bought an Italian convertible TR7 sports car, the Triumph dubbed "the shape of things to come." It cost a fortune, but I was making a fortune, and it drove faster than any car I'd ever dreamed of owning. I took to that car naturally, since my motorbike had required me to develop a real sense of balance and control. Rather than controlling a skinny little Java motorbike, however, I was at long last controlling a sleek and powerful machine that flew through the streets like a land rocket.

I was having so much fun. I was dating beautiful women, taking them to the best restaurants, buying the most expensive dinners, and drinking the most expensive wines and champagnes, and loving every minute of it. I felt like a prince, and still in my twenties, I was in no hurry to give up such a life.

It was right around this time that I went to a birthday party where I met a young man named Hadi. Hadi was half Indian and half Portuguese, and since my mother's family was of Portuguese descent, I felt an immediate affinity with him. Like me, Hadi had a real entrepreneurial streak. When he was fourteen or fifteen he had begun buying things at flea markets in Lisbon and bringing them to London, selling them for double the price. Talking with Hadi, I recalled the little cafeteria business I ran at that age and felt such an immediate connection with him.

Hadi had no formal education to speak of and could not write well, but he was the most street-smart person I'd ever known. As we got to know each other, I marveled at his business sense, and his spirit was so alive, it was contagious.

Soon Hadi and I were hanging out together regularly. On Wednesday nights we, often with other friends, might take the boat across the English Channel to the French port of Calais. From there we'd jump on a train to Paris or Berlin or whatever city might strike our fancy, and by Sunday we'd return, exhausted but exhilarated and ready for work the next morning.

How we had the energy for such a life I cannot imagine, but we were young and full of adventure. Still, we were both focused far more on our careers than on our adventures. Since I had a steady income and Hadi wanted to launch his own business, I helped him with some money, which he invested in his own kiosk business. It was a wise investment on both our parts, as now, years later, he is still my close friend and owns a fleet of kiosks, drives a Rolls-Royce, and travels the world in comfort and luxury.

Which is all to say that although I was not at all careful with my money in those early days, I chose my friends with care and learned that investing in the future of others brings me more joy than the finest fast car or fanciest clothes—though I like those, too! But as with all youthful indulgences, blowing my money was not something I intended to do all my life. I'd had a taste of adventure, but I also had goals. It was time to get serious about the direction of my life.

I worked for Sir Gray for the next few years, and while I was living the fast life, I had never left my Christian convictions. I had joined a Catholic church, and though I did not go to service regularly, I still prayed at least twice a day, and I felt my connection to God grow deeper each year. I had been sharing my money with others, and now I was reaching a point in my life where I wanted to share my connection to God with others. If I could help just one person grow closer to God, I figured, I would do far more for them than helping just with money. I would help their souls—just as my own soul had been shaped by the many generous people who'd appeared in my life, starting with my mother when she opened the world of God to me through St. Anthony's Shrine.

After I'd been working in London for a few years, this spiritual quest began to gnaw at me as my youthful life receded. I was maturing and seeking something more than sheer entertainment. I had joined forces with a Scottish Christian group, and they invited me to join them on a mission to Africa, which sounded like the most exotic and fascinating place I could imagine. I took a leave of absence from the hospital and planned to spend ten months in a town called Enugu in Nigeria.

In 1979, when I arrived in Enugu, the town—now a fairly large city and the capital of the Enugu state—was rather primitive, compared to London, which I had already grown so accustomed to. In many respects it reminded me of Kerala, with its shabby buildings, rusty corrugated metal roofs, and chaotic streets, but without the color and life of my home in India. The only color seemed to come from the earth, which was a reddish brown, the color of terra-cotta, but even this color was washed away by the dusty yellowish gray of the sky. The whole city was comprised of low buildings packed close together, the highest being the Hotel Presidential at seven stories. These buildings were encircled by a wreath of low mountains, giving it the feel of a dilapidated island in the middle of the vast continent of Africa.

While I found the town a dispiriting one, my purpose there pre-cluded fixating on the environment in which I'd found myself. I was there to heal people, and more importantly, to help them to heal themselves. We were promoting a public health campaign focused on teaching people how to avoid malaria by sleeping under mosquito nets treated with pesticides, as well as teaching them proper hygiene and training nurses and pharmacists how to use antibiotics to reduce infection.

I had all sorts of ideas in my head about how easy it would be. We would go down there, explain how to avoid these illnesses and infections, teach basic public health, and they would be so thankful that they would adopt all our suggestions and public health projects and get healthier. And hopefully, they would open their hearts to the word of God.

Well, let's just say it wasn't that easy. Half the time no one showed up, and when they did, they generally just wanted us to give them money. They might nod and say they'd use the nets and use the soap and boil the water before drinking it and that sort of thing, but then they'd go home and do none of it. It was incredibly frustrating. As for opening their hearts to the word of God, most of them were Muslim, and we were not allowed to promote Christianity as well as we would have liked. We tried to pray with them, but it was futile. Resigned to the futility of our efforts, I mostly focused on practicing medicine, seeing as many patients as I could and treating them. I saved many lives and had a good experience in many respects, but I never fully engaged myself there, and after seven or eight months I was ready to leave Nigeria behind and return to England.

After returning to England and working again with Sir Gray, I fell into a routine that was making me restless. I was growing less engaged in my work, and Sir Gray seemed to notice. One day he said to me, "I feel very bad, Lenny, but the truth is, I can't advance you any further. You've already reached the top here, but I think you should go further. I think you should look at other options."

His words were a blow, yet the idea was nothing I hadn't been considering myself. I was at the top of the managerial hierarchy, and I could remain there for another ten years or more, or I could use those ten years to excel even more.

"I could put you in touch with some connections I have in Australia or the United States," he suggested, "and I have great connections in the Middle East. There's a nice new hospital in Jeddah opening up, and they want British-trained doctors with the MRCP so they can treat the royal family of Saudi Arabia."

Of course, given my father's work in Yemen and that amazing year I'd spent there, I had a soft spot for the Middle East. So I agreed to give it a try. "Okay, I'll take a look," I told him. "I hate to leave you, but you're right. It's time I strike out and reach further."

Sir Gray was pleased, and while I felt a slight disappointment at the thought of leaving England, and Sir Gray, I knew that what lay ahead was an even greater adventure.

Sir Gray was true to his word and soon arranged an appointment for me as chief medical officer of the new hospital in Jeddah. I was offered an astronomical salary—several hundred thousands of dollars, tax free, and that was in the seventies. It was like being offered a million dollars a year these days. I'd never imagined earning such money. But it was nothing unusual for Saudi Arabia, as they had so much money and they paid all their doctors well. And Sir Gray was right. It was a great hospital, with state-of-the-art technology, the best-trained doctors, just a beautiful space. It had everything. Everything except life.

There was no social life, no drinking and no dating. There weren't young people to interact with, no educated people to talk to anywhere. And it was all desert. A TR7, the sports car I owned in London, was the hottest thing down there and so fast it ran in championship races—but there was no place to drive it in the desert, or more accurately, no point in driving it. Despite the opportunity for my career, I knew right away I would not be satisfied living there.

There was just nothing to do but work, and while the money was amazing, I had been living in England for nearly five years, and I was used to British life. I just couldn't imagine staying there a whole year.

There was something else as well. A big red flag. There were no churches, only mosques. I wouldn't have been able to pray in public or congregate openly with other Christians. That was a line I simply would not cross. I would not deny my faith. Given these factors, I did not take the job.

I didn't know what to do. When I shared my reticence with Sir Gray, he was understanding and got in touch with some of his colleagues in Australia, who offered me a few positions. While each was an impressive offer, Australia felt too remote, and I was at a loss as to what to do. I sank into such despair that I even thought about returning to India, where I could establish my own hospital. Then I did what all young men do when they don't know which direction to go—I called my father.

"Lenny," he said, "I think you have a lot of good skills. If you ask me, I would want you to come back home, but that's probably not what you want to do."

I agreed, but what were my options? Remain in England doing the same thing and going nowhere? And the truth was, I was growing weary of the wild nights and frivolous lifestyle, as much as I loved it. I sure didn't want to give it up altogether, as I would have to if I went to Saudi Arabia, but I was close to thirty and at a crossroads in my life. I didn't want to live in Saudi Arabia, but as much as I'd been relishing the bachelor life in England and my career in medicine working under Sir Gray, I never felt British. No matter how much money I made, I was still an immigrant. I was still the dark-skinned doctor who knew that this was not his place. Sure, I was at the same level as the wealthy White people I socialized with, but deep down I felt different. I had felt different even in India. I just didn't know what to do or where to go.

Then my father gave me an interesting piece of advice. "If they eat snake, you should eat the middle piece."

"What are you talking about?" I asked my father, bewildered. "You know I hate snakes!"

My father chuckled. "What I am telling you is wherever you go, whatever culture you go to, you must fit into that culture. You should be prepared to do what they do. Don't stay outside the culture. Don't be a foreigner all your life. Step inside the system."

My father was wise. He was telling me that if they served me snake, eat it with happiness. Eat the middle piece—embrace it.

With my father's advice in hand, I continued working with Sir Gray. I shared with him my desire to find a suitable position, one that would take me far but not strip me of any life at all, as Saudi Arabia would.

"Okay, then," he said, quite satisfied, as if he was finally certain of his diagnosis. "Let's look at the USA."

America. Yes, I would go to America. I had always dreamed of going to that magical land of opportunity, the world of *Life* magazine, *Reader's Digest*, and Voice of America. But first I'd wanted to know the British people and British spirit. Now, with that done, it was time to move on to my ultimate destination.

Now someone was offering me that opportunity. Like an angel guiding me toward my destiny, Sir Gray had opened a door to the land of my dreams.

✆ CHAPTER 7 ✇

Failures in Pursuit of Success

"What would you say to helping Thomas Starzl set up a new transplant program in the States?" Sir Gray asked me. Dr. Thomas Starzl's reputation preceded him—he was an amazing surgeon who had performed the first human liver transplant at the University of Colorado. Although organ transplants were still in their infancy in 1981, Dr. Starzl played a leading role in our understanding of organ rejection, and I was aware that the liver transplant program he developed at the University of Colorado was the most advanced in the world. "He's leaving Colorado to take his program to the University of Pittsburgh," Sir Gray told me, explaining that the medical school there offered even greater resources and opportunities. But what did I know about organ transplants? I'd never even performed surgery. The suggestion was flattering, but I wasn't sure it would be a good fit.

"Okay," I said, not wanting to reject another opportunity, for Sir Gray had already done so much to help me. "That is a good idea, but I can't go straight to the liver transplant program. I've never done surgeries before."

"That will not be a problem," Sir Gray assured me. "Organ transplants involve far more than surgery. It's a complex process that involves teamwork, and the program he's setting up will involve a broad system of medical resources and specialties."

That information changed the possibilities before me markedly. Being a part of a revolutionary medical team would be an amazing opportunity, as long as there was a fit for my skills. Giving the matter some thought, I realized that if there wasn't a good fit, I would create my own place in this new program. I looked at Sir Gray and smiled. "Then I'm in."

And with that, Sir Gray wrote to the University of Pittsburgh, and before long, I was accepted to join the program at the university's Montefiore Hospital—as soon as I'd passed my exams qualifying me to practice in the United States.

As I studied for my exam and prepared to move to Pittsburgh, I continued working for Sir Gray and began going to church more often and participating in various church activities. Though my work kept me so busy that I was still unable to attend services regularly, I continued with my devotion to God through twice daily prayer.

I also continued to see Hadi regularly. Our travel days behind us, we were both now laser-focused on our work, and I was feeling the first stirrings of desire for a more settled life.

Since coming to London I had seen and dated some beautiful women from many different countries in Europe, and many of them were quite wealthy in their own right, but in the back of my mind, I wanted to marry an Indian girl because I knew that would make my parents happy. I had grown up with the expectation that my parents would arrange my marriage for me, but as my life took on a direction all its own, it became clear that so too would my marriage. If my parents couldn't choose a bride for me, I wanted to at least honor them by marrying an Indian woman, one who would share my cultural background and language, and that meant returning to India.

It was during this period of reflection on my future and awaiting my move to Pittsburgh that a distant cousin of my mother's sought me out in London. He was a very distant cousin, the cousin of a cousin of a cousin or something on that order, but he knew of me through social connections and he had come from the same region in Kerala, so we shared common roots.

As we spoke, he seemed to be quite charmed and impressed by me. He introduced me to an Indian family who had emigrated from Zambia. There, I met Etna.

Etna was a young Indian woman with an undergraduate degree from the University of London and was completing her master's degree in architectural design at the University of California, Berkeley, in the United States. I found her to be an attractive, exceptionally bright young woman. She was quite friendly, with a bubbly personality that attracted me immediately. We went out a couple of times, both of us knowing that the objective of our dating was with the expectation that we might be suitable marriage partners.

A few months later, after she'd returned to the States, Etna got in touch with me and invited me to visit her in San Francisco. I had never been to America, which had been my dream since reading *Life* and *Reader's Digest* and listening to Voice of America, so I jumped at the chance. It just so happened that I was between my six-month rotations at the hospital, so the timing couldn't have been better. I flew to California and was impressed by the wealth and sophistication of America, but also by how nice everyone was. It was a marvelous time, and it was one of the only times in my life when I wasn't working. I knew then that life in America was just as I'd imagined it would be, and I wanted to make it my home. I also knew it was time I settled down and married. By the time I returned to England, Etna and I were engaged.

Under Indian custom, the bride's family would have paid for the wedding, as well as provided me with a considerable dowry reflecting my own status. Indeed, that was the case with my sister, Gladis, when she'd married, and my parents had to forgo not just a considerable financial sum but their very own home. But I knew that Etna's mother, a widow, had little to give, and I was in no need of a dowry.

I was just happy to marry an attractive young woman, and one who came from southern India and who, like me, was a Catholic. Consequently, I did not ask for any dowry and paid for the most elaborate wedding imaginable. High-ranking ministers, even the chief minister, the governor of the state of Kerala, attended the event, which was the flashiest wedding in the city. We spared no expense, filling the church and reception hall with tropical flowers and festive decor and feeding our guests with the most delicious food—and, of course, the freshest fish! It was a spectacular event, and both families were thrilled with our union.

By the time we got to the Taj Mahal for our honeymoon, however, I knew I'd made a mistake. What was intended to be a romantic start to our marriage instead illuminated the differences in our characters that would prove to be insurmountable. We both realized we were incompatible in spirit, but we had married, so we set out to make a life together.

We returned to London, where Etna had agreed to live until I'd passed my medical exam for practicing in the States and I could begin my residency in Pittsburgh. She had taken an extension on her graduate studies, and though she knew London well as she had lived there and her mother was still living there, once we were settled in, she decided to return to the States to continue her graduate studies. I suggested that she wait for me to start work, but eager to finish her graduate degree, she returned to San Francisco while I remained in London and continued my work.

It was right about this time that I went to Bristol to spend the weekend at the beach. As I was returning home in my TR7 with the top down, I noticed through the fog a pair of red lights in the distance. Though I thought there was plenty of time to stop, I was wrong. I crashed into a car—and three more cars ahead of it—all of which were waiting at a stoplight. All four cars had significant damage, and my car was totaled. Far worse, several others were hospitalized, but I walked away without a scratch. I had been spared by God once again. And once again, I knew that God had spared me for a reason. There was something God had planned for me, and I sensed I'd know it soon.

In the meantime, the insurance company bought me a brand-new TR7, and I was on the road again.

PART III

A SERIES OF FIRSTS

"Take the first step in faith. You don't have to see the whole staircase, just take the first step."

Rev. Martin Luther King Jr.

❧ CHAPTER 8 ❧

Marriage, Divorce,
and the American Dream

Imade the move to Pittsburgh in November 1981, and let's just say it was nothing like London. It was bitter cold, and while there were hills, they were more in the distance than in the city, which was dominated by industry. But aside from the initial impression that failed to impress me, I was excited to be living there. I would be spending most of my time at the university hospital, so I was unconcerned about the rest of the city, which was fortunately far better than living in Saudi Arabia. At least there was a social scene.

The first two weeks were difficult because I had to run so many errands and go through so much paperwork and get my license approved before I could start work. It was just one headache after another, and with no car and a freezing temperature unlike any I'd ever experienced, those two weeks were grueling. But I knew it was temporary, so I braved the snowy streets each day and took care of my business. In the meantime, I stayed at the YMCA, where the accommodations were rudimentary, but the proximity to the downtown area where I needed to do most of my business made the situation tolerable.

Once I had everything squared away and was cleared to work, the hospital gave me a modest one-bedroom apartment. It had none of the amenities of the London apartment—no laundry service, no food service, no housekeeper to keep the place clean—but it was connected by a tunnel to the hospital, which suited me just fine.

As for the hospital itself, in many respects it far exceeded the facilities in England. The diagnostic and computer capacities were amazing, and the research facilities were expansive. But I hadn't been there long before I realized that the heavy emphasis on research came at the cost of clinical care. Patient interaction was limited, with physicians spending more time analyzing lab results, consulting one another, or conducting research than having any actual hands-on treatment of patients, which was largely left to the nurses.

Fortunately, my experience in clinical care gave me an edge over the other residents. In one instance, we were all discussing the case of a patient who had been admitted for abdominal pain and diarrhea, and each resident assessed the medical records and gave their opinion—have this test or that, because it's irritable bowel syndrome, or Crohn's disease, or stress. Then came my turn.

"Order a barium enema," I instructed, "because I think this patient has colon cancer."

"And how do you know that?" the head physician asked, his voice conveying doubt at the foreign upstart who was so sure of himself.

"Because I met with the patient and felt his abdomen. I could feel the tumor."

For all the attention they'd given to scrutinizing the test results and medical notes, no one had thought to meet with the patient, much less to touch his abdomen. And sure enough, it turned out he had colon cancer. Such experiences became common as I focused more on clinical care and healing than most of my colleagues, who felt they were too busy and important to listen to their patients.

Meanwhile, having finished her graduate studies, Etna moved to Pittsburgh to join me, yet almost immediately she seemed to regret her decision. She absolutely hated the apartment, she hated Pittsburgh, and without work, she had little to keep her busy.

Our marriage was clearly off to a rough start, but by that point, I had already accepted that we had married in haste just to please our families, and ultimately, we were not suited for each other. I realized that I had made a bad decision, as had she, and it would be up to me to learn from that decision. In the meantime, I intended to keep my focus on my work and my life's direction.

By leaving England and coming to the United States, I knew that I would have to do my residency all over again, as is required in order to practice in the States. But after reviewing my professional history, it was decided that rather than do the normal three-year residency, mine could be cut to a year and a half. Unfortunately, Etna expressed she was unhappy with the prospect of living in Pittsburgh for even eighteen days, let alone eighteen months. There was nothing I could do or say to change her perspective.

A position had been cleared for me, personally. I had signed a contract. To abandon my position at such an early stage would have been a detriment to my career and all I had been working toward, as well as a slap in the face to those such as Sir Gray who'd opened doors for me. I was determined to stay.

After two or three months in Pittsburgh, I found Etna in the bedroom, packing her things. We'd had no argument; she was simply done with living in Pittsburgh and, apparently, with our marriage.

I didn't know where Etna was for about a month and presumed she'd gone to nearby Detroit to be with her sister, who lived there. Then one evening she called me out of the blue and told me she'd returned to California and that she was pregnant. She decided to have our baby in San Francisco, which left me with no options to participate in raising our child in any meaningful way.

As Etna and I went our separate ways and divorced, my work at the university was keeping me stimulated, as there was a great deal to learn. I was working my way up in the residency program by learning everything I could about liver disease. And because many of the people coming to us also had other chronic health problems, such as diabetes or obesity, that affect the functioning of the liver, and since I had so much experience working with such chronic health diseases, I was kept busy treating these patients.

While I was thrilled with having my residency time cut in half, I soon realized that all the other residents I was working with had come straight out of medical school. Right from the start I felt far more experienced than my colleagues, and my work demonstrated that fact. As my reputation grew, it seemed to expand exponentially, and soon I realized that I was sometimes admired even by accident.

It had so happened that the apartment they'd assigned me was in such an old building that the heat often went out. In Pittsburgh, the winters are bone-chilling, and an apartment without heat is more than just uncomfortable. It's near deadly. I didn't want to complain, and I felt it would be futile to do so, so on the nights when we had no heat, I would head down the hall to the hospital and look for an empty bed. If I couldn't find a bed, I'd camp out in the ER. Either way, I'd wake up at dawn when the food carts started clattering down the halls and head to the cafeteria, my clothes all rumpled and my face unshaven. It wasn't long before the rumors spread that I worked so hard I never even left the hospital. I decided to let those rumors circulate, as the truth—I had no heat in my apartment—seemed less impressive!

At any rate, after I'd been there six months, out of the nearly one hundred residents at the university, they selected me to be the chief resident the following year. It was a great honor, and I believe that in the university's 134-year history, I was the first foreign graduate they'd chosen for the honored position.

I was curious why I was chosen for such a distinct honor. Before long my curiosity burned and I needed to know, so I made an appointment with the head of the department who had made the selection. He was a world-renowned doctor from Harvard—a short man, astute, with an impeccable record. I sat before him alone and I asked him.

"Sir, I would like to know why you chose me for this coveted position," I said.

"Dr. Peters," he said. "I will tell you the truth. The doors are closed, so no one will hear us, and you cannot tell this to anyone."

I agreed.

"The first month you were here," he continued, "we gave you a cup of shit. You drank it so fast, we gave you a bowlful the next month. You finished that in no time. So we gave you a bucket. You enjoyed that also."

He told me I had consumed everything the hospital had thrown at me without a complaint and without hesitation, and I had solved each problem that came my way.

"That is why you are chief resident," he said. He smiled. So did I.

Unfortunately, with knowledge and experience often come resentments. Because I was writing up my medical orders in a style different from the way the nurses were accustomed, some of them, who were quite young, were upset. They wanted me to adapt to their way of doing things, rather than do things differently. So they began talking among themselves and decided to have their nursing manager speak with me.

One day the nursing manager, Janice, another pretty young blond woman with bright blue eyes and who was quite sharp, began checking up on me, asking how I was doing things and why, which I would patiently explain.

She was hanging around so much, in fact, that one day I asked her out for dinner. She agreed, and we went out and had a wonderful time. She told me that she had grown up in nearby Erie, Pennsylvania, and considered Pittsburgh her home. She also came from a good, Catholic, Polish American family. Her grandfather had started a business supply company, which her father had run until his retirement and then her brothers began managing it. I was impressed with this entrepreneurial background and the generational commitment to the family business.

Before long Janice and I were dating regularly and getting along quite well. Still, I was in no hurry for a commitment. But it wasn't long before I started to develop a taste for how it felt to be with someone who was a good fit, and that feeling was wonderful. I told Janice about my previous marriage, the divorce, and the baby on the way, but that didn't scare her off.

Not long after, Etna gave birth to a beautiful baby girl she named Shirin, but it was clear that I would play no role in her life. I considered the very real possibility that I might never see that precious baby but prayed to God that I would one day and that she would be safe. By that point I knew that Etna had a good heart and was a good person, but we would remain apart. Still trusting in the universe, I congratulated Etna on giving life to such a sweet child and continued with my work.

While the new residents were working hard until midnight, my years of experience served me well. I would finish my rounds much more quickly, being done with my work by late afternoon. After a while I was bored stiff once I got off work. I needed something to do. And I needed a car.

I missed my TR7 and had been walking or taking taxis since I'd gotten to the States. But I still hadn't recovered from the cost of moving to another country, as well as the wedding and divorce, so my finances were low despite my high income. I would have to secure a loan to buy a modest car until I could save up more money.

There was a branch of the Mellon Bank across the street from the hospital, so I went there and inquired about a car loan. After filling out the paperwork for a loan application, I met with the loan officer, a young, friendly man from Nebraska who seemed enthusiastic to help me. But his enthusiasm turned to regret when he looked over my application.

"I'm sorry, Mr. Peters, but I can't give you a loan."

I was astounded. How could I be a risk?

"What are you saying?" I asked him, incredulously. "I'm a doctor. I make a good income."

"I know," he said, shaking his head, "but you have no credit."

"Credit? What is this credit?" I asked him. I had never heard of credit.

He explained about credit and credit ratings, and I left, frustrated but not defeated. I returned a few more times, and each time it was the same answer. Eventually, he said to me, "You know, Dr. Peters, I like you. I'll tell you what. I'm going to be teaching an evening course on financial planning at the community college. Why don't you sit in on it? You'll learn all about credit and finance, and it will help you to manage your income."

I thought the idea sounded like a good one and agreed.

"In the meantime," he said, "why don't you apply for a credit card? That will establish your credit, and then you can apply for a loan."

Finally, I was getting somewhere. Credit card in hand, I began charging my restaurant meals and purchases and paid the bill promptly each month. Once my credit card had established the credit history I needed, I was able to get the $3,000 loan after all. I wasn't able to get much of a car with that, but I bought an old beat-up car that spent more time in the shop than on the road, but at least I had transportation. And with my divorce finalized, my relationship with Janice became more serious. She introduced me to Polish food, so we ate a lot of pierogi, soup, and cabbage, and I introduced her to southern Indian foods, so we ate a lot of spicy food. More importantly, we both shared a spiritual commitment. Although we were both born and raised as Catholics, we met a Presbyterian priest who we found quite interesting and began going to his church.

I met her family, and although her mother had passed away, her father, who had remarried, and I got along quite well. When I asked her to marry me, he not only gave me his blessing but he paid for a good-size wedding at their Catholic church in Erie. The wedding was a joyous one, as I was not marrying to please my family but because I'd found a partner I was confident was the right one for me.

We shared a love of medicine, we each had our own busy careers, and she was as excited as I was about investing in real estate. As we each also had an apartment, we decided our first investment would be our home. So once married, we were able to buy a small two-bedroom home in Squirrel Hill, an eclectic, mostly Jewish neighborhood with many small shops, bookstores, and the like. We were happy and ready to start a family.

I also began taking the banker's financial planning class, sitting in the back of the room, the oldest student in attendance. I attended to every word and learned more than I'd ever imagined I'd need to know about credit and financing. I also spent time talking with the instructor after class, asking lots of questions and impressing him with all I was picking up from his lectures. About halfway through the semester, however, he had a gallbladder attack and could no longer teach the class, so he asked me to teach the rest of it.

"But I can't teach a class on financial planning. I'm a student!" I protested.

"You just need to be one lesson ahead of the class," he assured me, "and you'll do fine."

So that's how I found myself teaching a class in financial planning while working as a resident during the day. By teaching the class, I discovered I was learning even more than I had learned as a student. And the more I learned, the more I realized that I could use my money to make more money. Still, despite my income, my savings were limited, so any investments I'd make would be limited as well.

One of the books I came across as I studied investments was a book by a man named Robert G. Allen. The book, *Nothing Down: How to Buy Real Estate with Little or No Money Down*, was already a bestseller, and his concept fascinated me. Allen suggested that property could be purchased directly from a motivated seller who owned the property outright and was willing to finance it himself in order to have a reliable income stream.

One of the ways to find such a property, he said, was to drive around town and look for For Sale by Owner signs. *Why not?* I thought. *Might as well give it a shot.* I have never gone through the front door for anything, it seemed, always finding my way forward by going through side doors or back doors. I'd invest in real estate the same way—by going through a back door.

So every afternoon or early evening after my shift, I would drive around town in my old jalopy, looking for For Sale by Owner signs. Whenever I found one that appeared to be put up by the owner and not a real estate agent, I wrote down the address and the phone number, and when I got home, I started making the calls. Nine out of ten never bothered to call me back, as I guess they weren't too eager to sell after all, but about one out of ten did.

Among them was an Italian man who owned a four-unit rental property. His wife was in a nursing home, and he wanted to return to Italy, but he needed some income to pay for her care. I met with him, and he liked me and saw that I had a steady income, so he agreed to sell me the property with no money down. And just like that, I was a landlord!

I had no skills in repair work, but having overseen the construction of my parents' house, I knew what to do. I hired people to paint and make minor repairs and was able to upgrade the building and rent it at a respectable profit. Having taken the financial planning course and grown a bit older and wiser, I knew better than to just blow my money. I set a new goal of investing the income I made into buying more properties, and it wasn't long before I owned four or five properties, all bringing me a steady stream of income—as well as appreciating year by year.

My life in Pittsburgh was moving remarkably fast. In just a few short years I had been made chief resident and completed my residency, I'd divorced and become a father, I'd remarried and become a landlord. I had even applied for citizenship, taken the exam, and eventually I became a U.S. citizen. Even better, it wasn't long before Janice was pregnant with our first child together, a daughter, Elise, born in 1985.

Meanwhile, Etna had graduated, and Shirin was growing up under her grandmother's care in London, where I could see her occasionally, however distant she may have been. While I would not be granted custody, I knew that Shirin was in a safe and secure home with Etna's mother, a kind, caring, and stable woman whom I respected.

Once again, God was looking out for me, and now, looking out for my daughter as well. Within a few years, however, my work at the university was no longer inspiring me. It was so difficult to get healthy livers delivered to us in time and in the proper condition for transplants. That meant that there just weren't enough transplants happening in those years to provide the professional opportunities I sought. Consequently, I decided to make the shift to internal medicine, specializing in gastroenterology, so that rather than wait any longer to get into the transplant field, I could excel in something I already had expertise in. I'd be working with the same livers, the same bile ducts, the same pancreases, but I just wouldn't focus on the transplant part. Life was good.

❧ CHAPTER 9 ❧

An Indian Immigrant
in the Old North State

As chief resident, I was in a good position to find a new job. Not only would my status make me an attractive candidate for upscale schools offering fellowships in gastroenterology to advance my training and skills, but I was the one bringing in visiting professors from other universities to give presentations to our staff. I would host their visits and get to know them—and they would get to know me. So once I had made up my mind to leave the University of Pittsburgh and began sending out my résumé and applying for fellowships, my network was sufficiently broad that I soon had multiple interviews and offers.

One of the most exciting was an offer from Harvard, and though I came close to accepting such a prestigious position, when I reflected on what my work would entail, I had to decline. Harvard wanted me to do 75 percent research, working in a lab, and only 25 percent clinical, which meant I would not be spending much time with patients. I was a healer. That meant I had to find a position where I could spend as much time caring for patients as possible. Fortunately, I hadn't been on the market long before I received an impressive offer from a renowned gastroenterologist, Dr. Donald Castell.

Don Castell was considered one of the premier researchers in the area of gastroenterology, with a remarkable career, having attended the death of John F. Kennedy, treated Secretary of State Henry Kissinger, and was now the chief of gastroenterology at Bowman Gray Center for Medical Education at Wake Forest School of Medicine in North Carolina. Don was recruiting people throughout the country to launch the new gastroenterology program at Wake Forest. Under his direction and given his stellar reputation in the field, there was no question it would be a state-of-the-art program in my field, and the opportunity to join his team was an incredible one.

I flew down to North Carolina, having never visited the South, and right away I was struck by how beautiful the area was. It was an up-and-coming region with affordable real estate, which meant it would be a good place to invest and an affordable place to buy a home. Even better, it wasn't nearly as cold as Pittsburgh.

I flew back home and shared my excitement with Janice. I suggested we go down there and give it a shot for two years. If we did not like it, we'd come back. She agreed, and in 1985, we sold our house in Pittsburgh and moved to North Carolina. We settled in Winston-Salem, tobacco country, where the air smelled like a freshly opened pack of cigarettes. I hadn't lived in such a lovely country atmosphere since I'd left India, and the bluish hue of the distant mountains, the rich abundance of trees and flowering bushes, and the many creeks and rivers that flowed through the city like lacework were a welcome change from the gray concrete and frigid winters I'd been living in.

We bought a nice two-story home and settled in. It wasn't long before we knew we weren't leaving. We loved it. But like all love, our move to North Carolina was not without its challenges. I was to discover that we were not just moving to another state—we were moving to another culture altogether.

It's no surprise that whatever I do, I tackle it with intensity, and my new position was no different. Once I was settled into my new job,

I encountered a clinical conundrum that got me to thinking. Once a patient comes to the emergency room complaining about chest pain, we don't know where that pain is coming from. It might be the heart, but it could also be esophageal pain, suggesting there is a problem with the esophagus. It all feels the same to the patient, and there was no diagnostic test at the time to help us determine what was going on.

Given that a portion of my job was research, our team decided to invent the diagnostic tool we needed. We got together with a fellow from the Ford Motor Company, an engineer, and we devised a little tube with pressure and pH monitors—in other words, acid sensors—attached to the tube. The engineer made a small box from something he bought at Kmart, put batteries in it, and connected it to the tube. It was a rather rudimentary contraption, but when we were done, we had a way to measure where the pain was coming from by inserting the tube into the esophagus, leaving it there, and every time acid came up, the sensors would note it. We also devised a way to record the measurements so that they could be reported to the health care providers.

The patient would record exactly when he or she had chest pain, and then the doctors could look at the recording, see what the recording showed, and correlate the patient's report with these objective recordings. We called it a twenty-four-hour pressure and pH monitor, and it was completely new. No one had ever made anything like it. There was just one problem. After we presented our monitor to some professors, they pointed out that we had no animal studies, so we couldn't test it on humans. And we couldn't test it on animals, because an animal couldn't tell us when it was in pain. It looked like we were at a dead end with our invention.

Then it came to me that it was time to find another back door. Like so many things in my life, I looked for the loophole. And the loophole was informed consent. You can test something without animal studies if the people you test it on are informed of what you are doing. Since the equipment wouldn't harm anyone, all I needed was to find some volunteers who would give their consent to try the monitor. But to find those volunteers, I needed to show that it was safe.

Standing before a roomful of my physician colleagues, I displayed my invention, then smeared some KY Jelly on the tube, and as they watched, I pushed the tube up my nose and down my throat.

"What the heck are you doing?" someone asked from the audience.

The room erupted in whispers as everyone turned to the doctor sitting beside him and wondered at the strange spectacle before them. Then I looped the remaining tube around my ear so it wouldn't be in the way, and for the next twenty-four hours, I carried the machine around, the tubing connected to it and, hence, to me.

Though I needed only three or four hours of recording, I wanted twenty-four hours of data, to demonstrate that anyone could tolerate the tubing and machine for that length of time. I walked around the hospital with it. I ate with it. I drove with it. I even slept with it. I wanted to be sure that everyone saw me living and working normally while recording valuable data. I may have looked odd, but the demonstration was a success. The university permitted us to test the machine on thirty patients, with their consent. It worked brilliantly for all of them. But it was hard work.

The machine measured a set of waves produced when the esophagus is squeezed, which it does three or four times a minute in normal cases. The bigger the wave, the more pain the patient is experiencing. This was before computers were commonplace and did these calculations for us, so in order to measure these waves, I had to record the measurements for twenty-four hours, manually measuring the height and width of each wave, then determine the average length and width of all the waves, and compare them to symptomatic stages versus asymptomatic stages. And I had to do that for every one of the thirty patients we were studying. It was mentally intense and incredibly time-consuming. I had to spend every weekend in the lab, on top of my regular hours, and it was just exhausting. But it produced the results we needed—the machine worked!

The next step in the scientific process was to publish our results. We wrote a peer-reviewed paper, listing me as first author, and had it published in the world's most prestigious peer-reviewed journal in gastroenterology—marking the first of many such articles I would publish in the field of medicine. The article generated a lot of buzz and was cited in countless other journals—the hallmark of a scholar's standing among their academic peers.

The invention was patented and the technology sold to a biomedical company for a significant sum. But because I had invented the machine as a university employee, alas, the university owned the intellectual property rights to that invention, so all the money went to Wake Forest. Nonetheless, I was thrilled. I was not just a doctor or a real estate investor. By the age of thirty-two, I had also become a successful inventor.

I enjoyed my job at Wake Forest and had learned more than I'd ever expected to learn. But inventing the monitor had made me realize that I didn't want to spend every weekend in a lab behind closed doors. I wasn't seeing the daylight, and I wasn't enjoying the nighttime. I was just there, working constantly. It was time for a change.

Initially, I thought I just needed to find a job with more clinical work. I wasn't alone in my frustrations with all the research, either. There were a couple of other physicians who felt the same as I did, and the three of us ended up on the job market at the same time, sending out application after application for a physician position in North Carolina.

One of the guys, a White guy, had no trouble finding a new position. Everybody wanted him. But the other physician, a Latino, was having the same experience I was having. Even though I'd never before had any trouble finding work, since moving to the South, I found that the job hunt was an entirely different game. I was not getting a good shake. I sent out application after application, and nobody was offering anything.

I didn't understand it. I was good. I was published. I had an excellent reputation, and I was clearly a hard worker. I'd even been chief resident at one of the major universities. I just wasn't getting any traction. Nor was my Latino colleague, himself an excellent physician.

The reason was becoming clear. I was a dark-skinned foreigner who spoke with an accent, and in the South, those traits branded me as unemployable.

I hadn't experienced any real racism in my life, at least nothing so blatant and extreme. As a Christian, I'd grown up as a minority in India, and I was a minority in England. But no one there had ever shunned me or refused to employ me.

I'd certainly had no adverse experiences in Pittsburgh, either. But the reality of the new Southern culture where I was raising my family was beginning to awaken me to the many obstacles before me for no reason other than my skin color and my accent.

Yet we had made friends in North Carolina, and we enjoyed it in so many ways. When I finally did receive an offer to work for a friend in San Diego and another one in Tampa, Florida, Janice and I realized that for all its racial divisions, we didn't want to leave. We'd grown to love the beauty of the region, the climate, the economic opportunities, and our friends. And it was a great place to raise children. So if we were to stay, I had to find another back door.

I thought about all the reasons I wanted to leave Wake Forest. I was working constantly, I had little control over my time, and despite having taken the job because there was less research than my other offers, I ended up having little time for clinical work.

I have always thrived on hard work, but if I was going to work that hard for the rest of my life, I didn't want to be doing it for someone else. I wanted to work for myself. I wanted to own my own time and my own intellectual property rights. I wanted to create something for my family that would last beyond me, something that I built myself and could pass on to my children and grandchildren.

I'd also learned a great deal about the economy and how investments and financing worked. I'd come a long way since taking the financial planning course. So after careful consideration, I decided I needed to do this myself.

I was taking a long walk, enjoying the gentle Southern breeze, as I contemplated the next step. I always had a plan. I had been percolating the next steps for some time. There was no reason to leave the South. There was a lot of investment potential in the South, which meant it was a great place to start a practice and for the kids to grow up.

At eighteen months, Elise was already walking and talking, and we were expecting our second child. Where we lived was no longer just about where we wanted to be. What kind of environment we could provide for our children was paramount.

I was going to have to find another back door. I decided to buy an existing practice because I didn't want to start my own and see just two patients the first day and three patients the second day. That would be a slow process and a risky one. But if I could buy a practice that was already established, I'd have twenty or thirty patients the very first day.

But at the back of my mind, I wrestled with my worries. Buying a practice would not just be costly, but it would be very, very risky. What if the patients fled when they discovered their doctor was a dark-skinned foreigner? I'd still owe for the practice but have no money coming in.

What's more, the technology involved in a decent practice is expensive and needs to be continually updated. What if I couldn't afford the best technology? For that matter, the malpractice insurance alone was exorbitant. My plan was indeed a risky one, but it was a risk I needed to take.

It is very hard to find a practice to buy, but I was not one to be discouraged by obstacles. I knew that God was on my side and would not abandon me at this point.

Someone is going to sell to me, I told myself with confidence. *I'm going to do something to make that happen. I'm going to find a lot of different people. The more people I can reach, the more possibilities I'll have.*

Just as I'd driven around Pittsburgh looking for a real estate investment, Janice and I found ourselves driving around outside the Winston-Salem area, looking for a practice.

We stopped at a phone booth and picked up spare phonebooks. Phonebooks are now a thing of the past, but back then, before Google and websites, phonebooks were where everyone's phone number was listed, and businesses posted their numbers, often with ads for their services, in the Yellow Pages.

We got the Winston-Salem phonebook and those for the outlying areas.

Once we got home, the task began. I wrote a letter inquiring about whether or not the physician might be interested in selling his business.

"Dear Doctor," my letter began, "I am a gastroenterologist at Wake Forest University with an interest in investing in a private practice and wondered if you might be interested in the opportunity to sell…"

I then had the letter photocopied and mailed to many practices. Then we drove to Greensboro and found more practices. Then we drove to High Point and did the same.

From the one hundred letters we mailed out, we received only about six responses. One of those responses was from a physician in High Point. I opened the letter from N. Hampton Chiles, M.D., an internist with a large and highly respected practice. Dr. Chiles explained that while he was an internist, he had trained in gastroenterology at the Mayo Clinic and was impressed with my background. In my letter I had noted my training and certifications, which included certifications in internal medicine, gastroenterology, and hepatology, so right off the bat we had common specializations.

Dr. Chiles indicated that he was interested in retiring in the near future and would consider selling his practice but would first like to meet with me.

I couldn't believe my good fortune. There weren't many people who had trained at the Mayo Clinic working in High Point, so I knew that his practice had to be one of the best in the city. I wrote back right away, and we arranged to meet one evening at his office, so that I could evaluate his practice—and he could evaluate me.

As I prepared for our meeting, I did some research on Dr. Chiles, and I learned that he owned the number one practice in the city, one where many millionaires went for treatment. He was a pillar of the community and very much a Southern gentleman. I wondered how he would react once he met me. Unlike applications for medical positions, where I included my résumé indicating I was from India, in my letter of introduction I had simply given an overview of my training in London and Pittsburgh. And with a name like Lenny Peters, there was no indication I was either a foreigner or dark skinned. But I was determined to win him over, regardless. He had a good practice and an interest in selling, and that's what I was looking for. I drove to High Point, my hopes high and my prayers strong.

When I pulled up to his office, I was surprised to see how modest it was in appearance. In stark contrast to its reputation as the premier medical practice in High Point, the building itself was a small brick ranch, quite a worn building, in fact. Prominently hanging outside, just as in an old-fashioned country doctor's practice, was a plaque reading N. Hampton Chiles, M.D., Medical Practice.

Although it was after hours, Dr. Chiles was expecting me, so I opened the door and stepped inside, calling out to him. A tall, regal man with gray hair who looked to be in his sixties stepped into the waiting room, and the shock on his face was unmistakable. He was clearly expecting a White man. For a moment he was at a loss for words, and I worried he was about to toss me out.

Unwilling to give him that chance, I gave him my warmest smile, held out my hand, and introduced myself. His momentary shock quickly turned to kindness, and after shaking my hand, he held open the door to his office and said, "Sit down, Lenny," motioning for me to take a chair.

His office was a simple but comfortable one, complete with a skeleton in the corner and an anatomical model of the nasal cavity on top of the file cabinet. His medical degree from the University of Louisville and certifications from the Mayo Clinic adorned the wall, alongside a striking Native American print of an eagle. Right away I could see myself sitting behind the desk, as he was, and making this practice my own.

As we spoke, it became clear that his initial shock notwithstanding, he was taking me seriously and treating me with the respect he would treat any White doctor. In the course of our conversation, I learned that in addition to his medical training, he was a Renaissance man of many interests, renowned not only for his medical knowledge but for his ethnographic study of Native Americans and a respectable indigenous art collection he had amassed over the years.

He explained that he and his wife, Amadine Griffin Chiles, a notable sculptor, were writing a book together on Native Americans, and the two of them had raised six children in High Point, each of whom was highly successful. Several were doctors, one was an attorney, and another, Lisa, was a high-ranking diplomat with the U.S. Foreign Service. She had married a man from Sri Lanka, and they were raising their children in Washington, D.C.—children who looked like my children. He was clearly a man who was comfortable around people from different backgrounds.

I felt as if I had met another divine soul sent by God. Here he was an aristocratic Southern White man, yet such an unconventional one. He was fascinated by other cultures, his son-in-law was from the same part of the world I was from, and his own grandchildren were nearly as dark as I was! What were the odds, I wondered, that of all the doctors I'd written to, he was the one who'd responded?

Within fifteen minutes of our meeting, Dr. Chiles leaned back in his chair, a big smile on his face, and told me in his honey-soaked Southern drawl, "If I sell this practice, Lenny, I will only sell it to you."

The moment he said that, I knew I had found my practice.

Dr. Chiles impressed upon me that although I had piqued his interest with my letter, he was hesitant to sell because while he knew he would be retiring soon, he wasn't quite ready to give up his practice altogether. He loved practicing medicine. I also realized that I had a lot to bring to him, because while he was clearly a country doctor at heart, providing the personal attention that people once expected of their physicians who treated them throughout their lives for all their medical problems, that old-school approach came at a cost.

Dr. Chiles had been trained to give excellent care to his patients, but he had not been trained with the state-of-the-art technologies that were revolutionizing internal medicine and gastroenterology, such as endoscopies. He offered barium enemas and upper GI X-rays, but patients had to go elsewhere for colonoscopies and endoscopies. But I could bring those innovations to his practice. So, after some talk back and forth about our mutual interests, once we'd eased from the possible stage to the probable stage of reaching an agreement, I spoke up.

"Okay, Dr. Chiles, that's great that you'd consider selling to me. I'd love to buy your practice. There's no ifs, ands, or buts about it. This is what I want to do. And I will do it, if not with you, with someone else. So if you're that person, we'll do the deal—and I hope it's you, because I like you. So, can we talk about some terms?"

I could see from his face that he was impressed with my candor. His smile was subtle but clearly approving. "Let's both think about it," he said, bringing our meeting to an amicable, if disappointing, close. "Let's meet again in a couple of days and I'll let you know what I think," he said.

I had no choice but to leave on a friendly note and wait anxiously over the next two days, praying to God that this arrangement, which I felt so deep in my heart was meant to be, would indeed, come to be.

Two days later, we met again at his office. "Lenny," he said, swiveling back and forth in his chair, contemplating what he was about to say, his gaze fixed on me. "Here's the deal. You pay me $250,000."

I nearly fell off my chair. Keep in mind, it was 1987, and I was only thirty-six years old by this point and raising a family. Sure, I made a reasonable salary, but a quarter of a million dollars was an astronomical sum, far more than I'd ever anticipated having to pay.

"And I will go to work for you," he said, "for at least two years, until I retire, at a salary of $120,000 per year. I won't do any administration—that's all yours. On day one, it's your practice and I'm your employee. It's all yours. You can change the name, do whatever you want. But that's what I want. It's been my whole life, and it means a great deal to me, so I want to know I'm leaving it in good hands. And I think you'd be just the person to take this over. I can see you're a good man and an excellent physician. I want to sell it to you, but these are my terms. Do you think you can handle it?"

A quarter of a million plus another quarter of a million over the next two years. Half a million dollars. Most doctors at my age would have half a million in annual salary guaranteed, with bonuses just to sign up, moving expenses, malpractice insurance, and health insurance all paid, all that on day one. And here I was presented with the opportunity to have half a million in debt on day one. It was not the career opportunity I had envisioned.

Like a crack in the universe, I felt my fantasies about owning my own practice split apart as I came face-to-face with the reality of the costs and the risks. I had not spent one day of my life in private practice. I had never run my own business. The most I'd ever done in that regard was buy some buildings and collect rents. Running a medical practice involved not just patient care, but purchasing equipment and supplies, paying salaries, paying taxes, buying insurance, sending out bills, collecting overdue bills, billing insurance companies, managing staff. It was an enormous number of things I would need to do to succeed, and up until now all I knew was medicine.

And on top of it all, this was a very White practice. As soon as those patients saw that Dr. Chiles had sold his practice to a man of color who spoke with a foreign accent, there was no question half of them would flee. And that would be if I were lucky. More probable, they'd simply toss me out of the city.

What had I talked myself into? I watched the reassuring gaze of Dr. Chiles. Through his eyes I saw his soul, sincere and generous but firm. There was no room for negotiation. Suddenly and with conviction, I said, "Yes, Dr. Chiles. I can handle it. We have a deal."

PART IV

ALWAYS A BACK DOOR

*"We are never defeated unless
we give up on God."*

U.S. President Ronald Reagan

❧ CHAPTER 10 ❧

Investing in Forgiveness

Since moving to North Carolina, I had been working far too many hours to focus on investing in real estate, but that initial investment of the four-unit building had proven to be the best one I could have made if for no other reason than it inspired me to invest in more buildings. Although I'd had little equity in the buildings when I'd first purchased them, as they appreciated over time, my equity had built up considerably, so that when I went to the bank to apply for a loan to purchase Dr. Chiles's practice, I was thrilled to be told that my loan was approved. How far I had come in just a few short years since I'd first asked a loan officer, "What is credit?"

Now I had credit—and considerable debt. I had no choice but to make that practice work. Fortunately, I knew that whatever obstacles I encountered would be knocked away by the sheer power of my work ethic. If there's one thing about me, it's that very few people can beat me in my ability to work hard. I may not be the smartest person in many areas, and I've gone head-to-head with much smarter people, but I'll beat them by working with an intensity they never imagined. And now I was going to be put to the test as I never had before—because if I couldn't repay that loan, I'd be broke. And that wasn't going to happen.

We sold our home in Winston-Salem and moved to High Point. We bought an even nicer house by a lake, where we lived with toddler Elise and our newborn, a son we named Anthony, after St. Anthony's Shrine. And by this point, my parents were aging, and although I returned regularly to visit them, I wanted them closer. My mother was thrilled with the idea, but my father was reluctant to leave his home in India. Nonetheless, my mother and I persuaded him to at least give it a try, and eventually he agreed. So our home was filled with the aromas of my mother's wonderful cooking and the laughter and joy of three generations living under a single roof.

My mother thoroughly enjoyed living with us, as well as the American way of life. My father, however, missed his friends and family back in India very much.

"I want to spend the rest of my life with my people in India," he said.

He decided to go back to India permanently. And as a devoted wife, my mother returned with him.

It was a nice neighborhood, with newer homes and many young families. Most of our neighbors were transplants themselves, coming from New York, New Jersey, and other Northern states, so we fit right in. We got together regularly, and our children played together. It was a lovely life for the most part. Yet still, I was an outsider professionally, and unlike in Pittsburgh and London, I didn't feel I was getting into the groove of things. I still wanted to break into the system, so to speak, to make my mark in the medical community, so as excited as I was with my new practice, I set my visions further afield toward an even better future.

Dr. Chiles and I had no legal document between us. We started to engage with lawyers, but eventually we decided to write on a piece of paper the six bullet points we agreed on, including the price. We both signed at the bottom and dated it, and we each kept a copy. That was all the legal documentation we had. For most people such an informal agreement over such a large investment would be laughable. For us, however, that document was sacred. We knew we trusted each other immensely and were drawn to each other by a magical bond and felt as if we had known each other in another life. Neither of us would cheat the other.

I started right off the bat with a staff of five, including Dr. Chiles. I was nervous about supervising someone so much my senior, especially in the practice that he had built, but he proved to be a man of his word—he saw himself as my employee from day one. It was on the first or second day that an incident occurred that made me see what a good and honest man he was.

The office manager noticed that the subscription for the Greensboro newspaper was coming up for renewal. It was a modest sum of only about twenty dollars or so, though the newspaper, which was left in the waiting room for patients, was for another town, so it really wasn't essential.

At any rate, she approached Dr. Chiles and asked, "Dr. Chiles, do we need to renew this paper or stop it?"

Dr. Chiles got up from his desk, stepped into the hall, and called out, "Where's Lenny?"

I popped my head out of my new office and said, "Yes?"

"That man is the boss," Dr. Chiles said, pointing to me. "I don't make any decisions. Whatever he says goes here. Everybody understand that?" He looked around at the small staff, who were watching the exchange.

All heads nodded.

That's when I knew everything would go smoothly with Dr. Chiles. It was just a small thing, a matter of only twenty dollars, but even in something so small, he had no problem giving up power.

Dr. Chiles was as generous with his patients as he was with his practice. Every patient who came into the office, whether a worker from one of the local furniture factories or a millionaire who owned one of the factories, he assured them all that I would give them the best care possible. And as for the vendors, the community leaders, anyone who had any influence, or whose products I might need to purchase, he told them all the same thing. "This is my son, Lenny. If I'm not here, I want you to take good care of him."

Nobody balked because Dr. Chiles wielded a lot of power in the community and was incredibly well respected. But I was no fool. I could tell they were wondering why he would pass on a good practice like that to a foreigner. Yet he never gave them the chance to express any prejudices. He stuck with me. And he worked harder than he had when he owned the practice himself. When he'd owned the practice, I was told he came in at seven o'clock every morning. But once he was working for me, he came in at six each morning and went straight to work, staying until six or seven at night. He was an amazing man, with a gentleness and a kindness few could match.

He also possessed a humility that I had not expected. Having trained at the Mayo Clinic, he had quite a reputation. Yet he hadn't kept up on the latest technologies and advances as well as I had, since I was more recently educated. Rather than resent me for knowing more about recent advances in medicine than he did, he wouldn't hesitate to seek me out for advice.

"How can I help?" he might ask, offering his services, or, "How is this done these days?" he might ask of a procedure, or "What can I do with this patient?" As I took over all the care, he gracefully stepped aside, not with shame, but with pride for having chosen someone he had complete confidence would give his patients the best possible treatment.

I came to see Dr. Chiles as someone the universe had sent to me just when I most needed him. Just as Mr. Joseph had entered my life when I so desperately desired a way to get out of India, or as Sir Gray had come into my life when I knew my only way to succeed in the United Kingdom was to practice in London, Dr. Chiles had come into my life by divine grace. I could not have succeeded without these kind souls, and it could not have been a coincidence that Dr. Chiles and I had found each other. I was able to free him from the responsibilities of his practice and provide him with a comfortable retirement, and he was able to confer on me the practice that would launch my own prosperity. I had no doubt that he had been sent by God.

For the first couple of months, however, no matter how much confidence Dr. Chiles had in me, the office staff was distrustful. They weren't too happy about working for this dark-skinned guy, and they were confused by having Dr. Chiles around while suddenly being expected to take orders from the foreigner. They still viewed him as the boss, even if he encouraged them not to, so there was some strain. They just didn't know what to make of me.

With all of us in the small office space, it was also quite cramped. At one point, the office manager, Sandra, said we'd need to bring in someone to do the billing, but she didn't know how to make that happen.

"Where's this billing person going to sit?" she asked. "There's no place to put them."

"I'm in the middle of patients," I told her. "Just give me a bit of time. I'll find the space." I returned to my work, all the while knowing that if there was a problem, I intended to find a solution. Once I had a few minutes between patients, I found Sandra and said, "Come with me. I'll show you where we'll put the billing person."

We walked down the hall, and I opened the door to the bathroom, which was just a closet with a toilet and a sink. I put the toilet lid down and said, "That's a good seat!"

Sandra looked at me as if I were cracked. But she knew me well enough by that point to know that while I would not put someone to work in the john, I'd made my point. We had to do with what we had, and if all we had was a toilet to sit on, that's what we would do.

Of course, we did hire someone to do the billing, and we did find a place to squeeze her in, and I even hired a physician assistant to help me. While it was certainly crowded, the point is, I started that practice in the same way I had gotten anything done in life—by working with what I had.

I worked incredibly hard that first year. I worked hard because it is my nature, but I worked even harder because I did not want to let Dr. Chiles down. Fortunately, I'd become quite efficient with time management and had always been a good planner. I focused on what needed attention and how quickly I could attend to that. I didn't dance around an issue, talk to lots of people for feedback, and then think it through. If I needed to make a decision, I made it with the information I had on hand. I didn't need to be right 100 percent of the time. I needed to be right only 80 percent of the time.

I ascribed to my own version of the 80/20 rule. The 80/20 rule suggests that 80 percent of our work is done in 20 percent of our time. In other words, while most of our time is squandered, if we focus on the 20 percent of our time where we are most efficient, we will get more done. I took that rule a step further, realizing that to get things done, I couldn't afford to spend a lot of time reflecting on what needed to get done. I had to just do it. I had to make decisions quickly and take action right away. My thinking is, if you are making correct decisions 100 percent of the time, you're not trying hard enough. You're only making safe, easy decisions. If you're making good decisions only half the time, you're not smart. But if 80 percent of the time you're making good decisions, it means you're pushing yourself hard enough to make those good decisions—and that means that 20 percent of the time you're going to be wrong. That's the way you learn. That's how you know you're growing and pushing yourself to the best of your ability.

I knew I was an 80/20 guy. Twenty percent of the time I blew it. I acted too soon, did not have the information that I needed. But 80 percent of the time I was right. I was a good planner and managed my time well. I worked long hours, but more than that, I was efficient. I knew what needed attention and how quickly I could attend to a problem. I didn't think through a bunch of different variables and then make the decision. If I needed to make a decision, I would make it with the information available to me. So with that thinking, I made decisions quickly, I hired good people without a lot of wasted time, and I got a great deal done.

I also worked so hard because I was afraid I would fail and I never wanted to return to poverty. I did not want to raise my children in the poverty I had been raised in, I did not want to disappoint my parents by failing in my business, and I did not want to put my future on the line. I had no choice but to succeed.

But there were those who wanted me to fail. There were only two other doctors of color in town, both African Americans, and they worked on the poor side of town. So here comes this young guy with dark skin, speaking with an accent, saying he was an Indian, which just confused the hell out of everybody. And I'm treating all White patients. Naturally, these two doctors had some resentment toward me, but they didn't treat me badly. They weren't any more supportive of me than the White physicians in town were, but unlike the White physicians, they didn't fight me. That may have been because they weren't powerful. But to the extent they did have any power, they were not going to let a dark-skinned foreigner succeed.

Once again, I needed a back door.

Just as I'd learned about racial prejudice when I moved to North Carolina, once I began working in High Point and had my own practice, I came to learn about prejudice all over again. Here, I was neither White nor Black. When people saw that I was the doctor, they just couldn't fathom it. Of course, more educated people could because they had met international students in graduate school. But the average working-class person was inevitably confused. The only thing they knew about India was that it was a place where everyone was starving—surely there couldn't be educated, successful people from such a place, they reasoned.

A common question I was asked was whether I was White or Black. If the person was White, I would say, "Yes, I'm White, but I lived in the Caribbean for many years and my skin got dark." That would seem to satisfy them that they were safe in my hands.

And if they were Black, I would say, "Yes, I'm Black. But I straightened my hair." And they would be satisfied that they were safe in my hands. Many knew I had a good sense of humor.

I would smile as I joked with them in this way, but inside I wasn't smiling. Inside it was gnawing away at me as I had to prove again and again my basic competence and humanity. But in order to succeed, I knew I needed to pack away those thoughts and push through them. I just had to keep going.

I could not allow prejudice to demoralize me. I had to hold my head high and use the power of forgiveness to overcome such challenges. I knew I could not win by throwing stones. I had to win them over from within and with kindness.

And I had to keep going even when the White doctors wouldn't refer their gastroenterology patients to me. Fortunately, my experience at Wake Forest had trained me well. One of the techniques I'd developed while working there was a method for cauterizing a bleeding ulcer using a new technology that few others knew how to use. If someone was throwing up blood, rather than rush them into surgery, which might mean waiting for a surgeon to arrive, I would sedate them and thread a tube through their mouth into their stomach and cauterize the ulcer without having to cut the patient open. It turned out I had to do this procedure several times, so it wasn't long before I had established a reputation as someone who could save lives. Patients began coming to me, telling me that their doctors had told them not to go to me, but they came anyway. Eventually, these doctors had no choice but to call me when they needed help, and my day would be spent working at the practice, coming home for dinner and a nap, then being called into the ER for various emergencies.

The racism remained, but I'd found a way to transcend that racism just by being so good at what I did that they had to rely on me. Yet, as much as I tried to transcend the racism I encountered by working hard and killing them with kindness, it distressed me to see the impact on my family. I decided I had to do something to hold my family together spiritually. We joined the oldest Presbyterian church in the city and had our children baptized there, we contributed generously, and we experienced no hostility. We did everything we could to fit in. We had a great church experience. I was determined that my new friends, neighbors, and colleagues would not look down upon me or my family. Instead, I was determined that they would look up to us.

It was a great, if difficult, year, and by the end of that year, after paying the staff, including Dr. Chiles's salary, I had made a profit. And that profit was more than one million dollars.

Even I was shocked at how well I had done, through nothing more than hard, hard work. But I knew that no amount of hard work and expertise would be enough, so by the end of the first year, I set my sights even higher. I decided I was going to build the nicest-looking medical building in all of High Point. The best one. One that would have the unmistakable stamp of my success on its facade. Just as I'd built Bethany for my parents, I would now build Bethany Medical Center—and I would make it the most successful medical practice in the region.

CHAPTER 11

Doctor, Banker, Real Estate Developer

We'd been working in such cramped quarters for more than a year, and every day it felt more cramped than the day before. I wanted space. Lots of it. As I left work and headed to my car each evening, I gazed at the street, imagining where I might build the medical center of my dreams. I envisioned a building of two stories, built of glass, with lots of light and lots of white. And marble inside and out. I wanted it to be so clean it would glisten. I wanted it to be the most striking and modern medical building in all of High Point.

At the top of the building, I would build a door—or more accurately, what looked like a door. I wanted to place my emblem on that door, to symbolize the door to our center was open to anyone. And anyone who came through our doors would be united through our love for our fellow human beings. Naturally, I would name it Bethany, just as I'd done with my parents' home. It would be a medical center open to all. The Bethany Medical Center. I wrote up my vision, explaining the mission of the center, framed it, and posted it in our office so that everyone who worked for me or came to us for treatment knew that we were focused on the future, and that future would offer the most advanced treatment available anywhere in the Tri-City region and beyond.

Right across the street, on Westwood Avenue, was an apartment building and four houses that had seen better days. The apartment building was old and shabby, as were the houses. They could not have been worth much, and the owners of the houses would probably like the idea of selling and moving to a better home. I got to imagining my medical center right there, where those buildings were, stretching the whole block.

Eventually, the image in my mind took hold, and I knew that I wanted to buy that block. I wanted to buy the apartment building and all the houses and transform the block from a dying one to a thriving one.

I looked up the property records on the apartment building and learned that it was owned by a trust, managed by the local bank, High Point Bank and Trust. One day, determined to buy the property one way or another, I met with one of the senior members of the bank, a prominent banker in town. He no doubt held a lot of sway in such a small town, so gaining his approval would be important.

After his secretary had told him a Dr. Lenny Peters was there to meet with him, her voice unmistakably wary, I was ushered into his office, where I extended my hand before taking a seat at his desk.

He took one look at me, and his face registered disapproval, while shaking my hand as if it were infectious. I could tell he thought he was wasting his time talking to some foreigner with skin as dark as a Black man.

"Yes, what can I do for you, Mr. Peters?" he asked, as if I were about to sell him a set of encyclopedias.

"Hello," I said, putting on my broadest smile and my greatest charm, "I'm Dr. Lenny Peters." I let the "doctor" sink in just a second before continuing. "I recently bought Dr. Chiles's practice, and I'm interested in expanding it. I understand that you manage the trust for the apartment building on Westwood Avenue, and I'd like to buy that building."

I might as well have told him I was interested in buying the bank itself. He was incredulous.

"No," he said, rising from his chair to bid me goodbye. "It's not for sale."

"Maybe it's not on the market," I said, making no move to leave, "but it is an investment. And that means if the price is a good one, you'll sell. I'd at least like the chance to discuss a fair price with you."

His eyes narrowed, and he gestured for me to leave. "It's not for sale to you. Good day, Mr. Peters."

"Dr. Peters," I corrected him. "And I'm sorry you feel that way. But I am going to buy that building." I fixed my eyes on him, letting him know I was serious. Then I left, unsuccessful but all the more resolved to buy that building, whatever it took.

Having taken the financial planning course, I had learned a few things. And one of those things I'd learned was that trust documents are public record. So I had someone go to the courthouse and find the trust documents for the building. I learned that the building had been inherited by two brothers who lived in Virginia and had put the property in the trust to protect their financial interests. I tracked down the phone number of one of the men and gave him a call.

"I want to buy your building on Westwood Avenue in High Point," I said after introducing myself. "Would you consider selling it?"

"Sure," he said. "Give me a good price."

We spent the next forty-five minutes negotiating a price and terms, and by the time I hung up the phone, I had an agreement to buy the building.

Once that agreement was signed and in my hand, I went to the bank and met again with the banker who had so summarily dismissed me. He had no interest in meeting with me again, but before he had a chance to insult me once more, I said, "I have an agreement. I'm buying that building, and I know it's illegal for a trust to block a sale. And I have the down payment, assets, income, and credit to secure a loan for the purchase price. If I don't get the loan from you, I'll get it from some-one else. But denying my loan on the basis of my race is also illegal. So, shall we talk here or in court?"

They sold me the building. But I was still not satisfied. I told myself I would buy his whole bank one day, and added that bank to my future vision.

The next step was to buy the homes on the block. I had no trouble buying the first two, and the last two, but the house in the middle of that row of homes was owned by an elderly woman who refused to sell. I wasn't going to look good if I threw an old lady out of her house, but I wasn't about to give up now that I had bought up everything on the block. So I decided not to worry about it for the time being and continue with my plans.

I found an architectural firm in Charlotte that specialized in med-ical architecture and was considered the best firm in the South. They came out, surveyed the property, discussed my vision, and drew up the plans. The strip where the houses were would be used for parking, but that house in the middle posed a problem. It blocked everything.

"Dr. Peters, you can't build a parking lot here," the architects told me, "not with that house right there."

Since I don't pay much attention to people telling me what I can't do, I just laughed. "What you're telling me is I can't go through the front door," I replied, noting the confusion on their faces. "I know what you're telling me, but I'm going to ask the same question again and again, until I hear what side door or back door we can go through. Don't tell me how we *can't* build it. Tell me how we *can* do it."

Finally, they got it. They put their heads together and came back with a solution. "What if we put the building on stilts and have the parking underneath the building? We can have an elevator lead to the main entrance on the second floor."

I thought about it a moment, smiled, and told them, "There it is. There's your back door!"

Within one year, the building was completed. Just two years after I'd moved to the city, I was ready to open the doors to Bethany Medical Center—the most impressive medical building in all of High Point.

As I was launching my new practice, I had noted how difficult it was for patients to get appointments with local physicians. It was not unusual for them to have to wait six weeks or longer just to see a doctor. In addition, because they closed their practices by 5:00 p.m., patients often had to take time off work, which could be difficult and costly. Consequently, I decided to keep my doors open from 8:00 a.m. to 8:00 p.m. seven days a week—and walk-ins were welcome.

That move alone brought the patients in droves, and we soon became the largest medical group in the area. With Bethany Medical Center up and running, however, I faced another challenge. Dr. Chiles's health was declining, and he was ready to retire. At just about the same time, my physician assistant announced that he was moving to Tennessee. I couldn't possibly manage all the patients myself. I needed help.

I began by looking for a new PA. A few months earlier, a young man from the Wake Forest Physician Assistant program had done an internship with me. His name was Don Bulla, and he had been born and raised in Asheboro, a town thirty minutes away from High Point. His family had been in the state for a couple of hundred years. Far from an outsider, he was a real Southerner, young, charismatic, and very loyal.

Since his internship, Don had graduated at the top of his class from the PA program and was a licensed physician assistant. I called him up, told him about my new practice, and jokingly said, "Don, I'll pay you half as much as anyone else, but I want you to work twice as hard. Is that a deal?"

Don's immediate response was "It's a deal. I like you, Dr. Peters, and I've already worked with you. I know what I'm getting into, and I'm on board."

That was more than thirty years ago, and Don, now vice president of Bethany Medical and president of Peters Medical Research, is still with me.

Meanwhile, the problem remained about the elderly woman's house. After a year of operation, her house was still there, but now she was surrounded by the bright lights of the parking lot and hospital. This was a reality we had already presented her with when we first proposed buying her home, yet she had held firm and told us she didn't care. She was quite friendly about it, but she said she wasn't going to move. While it may not have been a problem for her, it certainly was for me. It didn't look good having a house in the middle of our parking lot, so throughout that first year, I would have various Realtors talk with her, and every time they came back and said she wasn't budging. Finally, I'd had enough, and I said to myself, *There must be another way to do this.*

I found the number of a local bakery in the phone book and ordered a cake to arrive the next day. The following afternoon at three o'clock, with the cake in hand, I knocked on the door of the elderly woman, Mrs. Jones.

"Hello, Mrs. Jones. I'm Dr. Peters, the owner of the Bethany Medical Center. Do you mind if I come in?" I held out the cake to her, watching her eyes widen but her posture stiffen.

"Yes, I know you," she said, taking the cake and ushering me inside. "But I'm not selling my house."

"I didn't say I wanted to buy your house, Mrs. Jones. I just wanted to bring you a cake."

She was clearly delighted at the offer and, I suspect, the company, and gestured for me to take a seat. "You know, Dr. Peters," she said as she slowly eased herself into her chair, "I've been meaning to come and see you and the other doctors in your clinic. I have this arthritis. I have a real problem going up and down stairs, and my bedroom is upstairs. It's gotten so it takes me half the night to make it to bed these days." She laughed, but I didn't doubt for a minute that her pain was real.

Moreover, she was telling me exactly what I needed to know—why her house wasn't a good one for her anymore. As I looked around the house, it was clear that it was well loved—filled with her personal mementos and tastefully decorated from decades past. Cracks in the walls told me the foundation was going, while worn carpeting, a broken front window, and a poorly patched leak in the ceiling made it clear she didn't have the money to keep it up.

"It sounds like it's gotten hard for you to get around," I said, expressing my empathy and echoing her concerns.

"It sure is. I'm getting older. I could fall and break my hip."

"I sure wouldn't want that happening to you, Mrs. Jones. I see a lot of patients who've had falls, and it's not something anyone wants. It sounds like you might need to get a one-story house so you don't have to climb any more stairs."

She smiled mischievously and shook her finger at me. "Now, Dr. Peters, you aren't fooling me one bit! I told you I'm not selling my house, and you're not going to talk me out of it just because you brought me this beautiful cake!" She laughed, so I knew I was still in her good humor. Then she went on. "Besides, if I sell this house, the government will take half of that as tax, because I don't owe anything on it. I own it outright. If that happened, I'd end up with only half as much money and no house. I couldn't buy anything with that."

So the problem wasn't that she wanted to keep living in the house. If anything, she wanted a more suitable house. The problem was that she was concerned about taxes. Just as I'd suspected, nobody had ever sat her down and talked to her to find out what she wanted. Everyone had approached her by telling her why I wanted to buy her house, not asking why she didn't want to sell it.

"You know what?" I said. "I have an idea. How about if I just buy you a house with two bedrooms on one level. Brand-new. Then I will give you that house, and you will give me this house. That way you won't owe any taxes. It's called a 1031 exchange."

Her eyes widened even more than when she'd seen the cake. "Would you do that for me, Dr. Peters?"

"Of course I would," I said. "If the only reason you're concerned about selling is that you'd owe too much on taxes, then let's just find you a nice house you'll like and trade, so you don't have to pay them."

"Dr. Peters," she said, as the glow of youth seemed to return to her face, "we have a deal. How about celebrating with a piece of that delicious cake?"

And that's how I ended up acquiring the whole block. As for Mrs. Jones, I bought her a one-level house in a new development right next to her church. The value was about the same as the value of her house, which I tore down. Once it was torn down, I was able to close off the bottom floor that had been used as a parking lot and make it into the first floor, giving me the two-story building I'd set out to build.

After Dr. Chiles's retirement, Don and I had formed the nucleus of the practice at Bethany Medical. Right from the start, Don proved to be another one of the people sent by divine grace because he worked the same long hours as I did. He would arrive even earlier than I did and leave even later, and he made his rounds with an expertise and care that endeared him to our patients. We made an excellent team, and his Southern roots helped legitimize Bethany Medical in the community. As the practice grew, however, it became clear that even with Don's expert assistance, I needed another doctor.

When I had first moved to High Point, there was one other gastroenterologist in town, and he wanted me to join him—I suspect because he wanted to prevent me from going into competition with him, not from any genuine desire to have me join his practice.

Because Winston-Salem and High Point are so close, I had already learned of his reputation because I'd treated many of his patients, and I knew he wasn't particularly skilled. I wasn't comfortable joining him, as I didn't want to be affiliated with his work, which I found inadequate, so I had declined. As a result, he never said a kind word to me.

He always treated me badly, and I have no doubt he wasted no time in denigrating me to other doctors in the area.

My growing success with Bethany Medical Center was not being well received by my other medical colleagues in the area, either, despite my affiliation with Dr. Chiles. I wasn't getting any referrals from prominent White doctors whose patients needed to see a gastroenterologist, even though I had established a great practice in the city. When I'd ask these doctors about it—seemingly friendly colleagues to my face—their typical response was "Well, they just don't want to go to your center." What they didn't know, though, was that their patients *were* coming to me—and asking me not to tell their doctors.

But I did tell them. I wasn't going to let them continue to smear me to their patients, and I wasn't going to treat my patients in a clandestine relationship as if I were some kind of quack. Instead, I'd go straight to those doctors' offices and confront them. "This patient of yours came to see me," I'd say, showing them my notes, "but you told them not to see me."

Their inevitable denial would come. "Oh, I never said that." But their faces belied their duplicity.

My skills were undeniable, however, and by word of mouth and my open-door policy, my practice continued to grow. But I knew that didn't mean it would continue to do so.

I realized that as long as I was dependent on their referrals, I was facing an uphill battle. They made it very difficult for me. They ultimately wanted to drive me out of the community, so they would continue to tell their patients who needed to see a gastroenterologist not to come to me. The only way I could succeed would be to expand my practice by offering more specialties, which meant expanding the specialists we had on staff. I also realized that I would have to recruit new physicians to my practice.

I was building this practice myself, and I intended to remain in control of it. But I did need to attract good doctors, so I offered them good income, benefits, and good work hours.

Since I had a good hand on gastroenterology and internal medicine, I considered what other specialty I should add. I assessed our patient needs and realized I could use a pulmonologist, someone who specialized in lung disorders. Not only were we living in tobacco country, but there were rising rates of asthma and respiratory disorders among both children and adults, and having someone who could address such chronic diseases would help us to stand out. Wanting to recruit nationally so I could hire the best pulmonologist I could find, I advertised in the major medical journals.

It wasn't long before I got a call from someone finishing up at the medical school at UCLA. He told me he was from South Carolina, where his father was a police officer and his mother was a teacher. Right off the bat, that told me two things. First, he was a Southerner. That was good. Second, he was the first in his family to get an advanced degree—that meant he was a hard worker. And while he wanted to return to the South, he didn't want to be too close to his parents, so he was likely to stay. He was a great candidate, so I invited him for an interview.

When he walked through the door, I was surprised to see that he was African American. I immediately felt a kinship with him as another physician of color, yet I knew hiring a Black man would not go over well, because he was going to be a critical care specialist. It was a powerful position because every patient who was sick in the hospital would have a consultation with him—which meant that all the doctors would have to go through him when their patients got sick. And I'd been in North Carolina long enough to know that most of the doctors did not want to work with Black doctors.

But as far as I was concerned, he was the best choice. I'd interviewed others for the position, and this man was the most qualified of them all. So I decided I'd take the risk. I didn't care at all what color his skin was. I wanted the best doctor I could find, and he was the one. Yet even though I was becoming accustomed to the racism in the South, I was wholly unprepared for the backlash that followed when I hired a Black physician.

Oh my God. The whole place erupted. The glares. The comments. The presumption that he wasn't qualified. The presumption that he was hired not because he was the best but because he was Black, the implication being he was less qualified and that he'd taken a White man's job. All that was to be expected, however. What I was to discover was that the glares, comments, and assumptions were the least of it. My phone started ringing with anonymous callers threatening my business, threatening me, and most terrifying of all, threatening to hurt my children.

I was furious. I had hired the best physician I could find, and these men claiming to be God-fearing Christians were acting quite the opposite. I prayed for patience, for tolerance, for forgiveness. But mostly I prayed for the safety of my family.

One thing I wasn't going to do, however, was leave town. No, I was going to show them that I could not be intimidated.

Instead of firing my pulmonologist, I placed an ad for another pulmonary critical care physician. This time, however, I was going to hire a White doctor, not to appease the troublemakers, but to show them that White doctors and Black doctors could work side by side. It was going to cost me some money, but it would demonstrate racial integration at work. Patients would see a White guy one day, a Black guy another day, and they would discover that they received the same care by a racially integrated physician partnership.

I found just the physician I was looking for, right out of Stanford. A Stanford- educated physician is not cheap, and I had to pay him a lot more money than the other one, but once he was on board, the calls quieted. Even better, the patients began to respond just as I'd hoped. They saw us all working together, me—the Indian with the funny accent—the Black doctor, the White doctor, and the White Southern PA. Unfortunately, however, the White doctor didn't work nearly as hard as the Black doctor, but his work was good, and the decision to hire him had been a good one, particularly in light of the ongoing problems I was having gaining acceptance with the broader medical community in High Point, where anyone who hadn't been in the area for generations was unwelcome—especially if they were successful.

The greater my success, the greater my visibility, and the greater my visibility, the more problematic they found me to be. That was fine with me. I was happy to be their problem. It meant I was succeeding.

There were a number of different groups of doctors operating under various practices and clinics. The hospital helped them to form a single, united group called Cornerstone Healthcare, comprised of about two hundred doctors, to compete with me and to restrict my growth.

If I were recruiting a doctor, I was out of luck when it came to touring the hospital—I would not receive any help, and they would badmouth me any way they could. Once Cornerstone was formed, I had no way to make progress. The hospital was hitting me from one end, and Cornerstone was hitting me from the other.

I had nowhere to turn but to God. "Good Lord," I prayed, "why are they doing this to me? Why did you bring me to High Point? I have been to London, Pittsburgh, even San Francisco—I could have gone anywhere to work. Why did you bring me here?"

I prayed this prayer each day and each night, and then one day, I heard a voice. It said, "Say a prayer."

"Okay, I'll pray," I said, and I started praying even more. "Okay, God, I'm praying. And they're still hitting me. Why are you putting me through all of this?"

The voice replied, "Pray as I taught you, as I taught you to pray."

I understood what that meant. It was what my mother taught me as a child at St. Anthony's Shrine in India—to be on my knees and bend my forehead until it touched the ground, my arms crossed over my chest in prayer. I was to bend down in supplication, to fall down on my knees in prayer. I got down on my knees, lowered my head, and started praying, lowering my head even further until it touched the floor, and

I drew on all my emotion, all my passion, to pray as strongly as I'd ever prayed.

And as God has always done, He answered my prayers. Shortly after, it was discovered that the Cornerstone deal had cost the hospital far too much money. The group was draining revenue from the hospital, while Cornerstone was reported to be $29 million in debt. The administrator resigned, and Cornerstone went bankrupt. The hospital was sold to the University of North Carolina, Chapel Hill, and four years later, sold again to Wake Forest University. When the carnage was over, I emerged from my prayers and was lifted up. Bethany became the largest independent health care provider in the Triad.

I felt the need to celebrate. I went to the nearest Rolls-Royce dealership and asked to see their biggest car.

The dealer was an acquaintance of mine, but when it came time to conclude the transaction, he invited me into a nearby office to discuss the financing options. I held up my hand, indicating he could stop. "That won't be necessary," I responded. "I will pay cash."

With that I pulled out my checkbook and wrote a check for the full amount.

He said the deal would have to hold a day or two until the check cleared, but I did not mind. I thanked him and drove away in my red Ferrari.

A few days later I was driving around town in the biggest, bluest Rolls-Royce I had ever seen.

The message was clear. They could shun me all they wanted, but I wasn't going anywhere.

Those early years were hard, but by the time I was forty, I was worth millions, and soon after I was driving not just a Rolls, but also a Porsche and a Ferrari. I had it made.

But the racism hadn't stopped. There were still those who looked down on me. It was time to make it clear that I wasn't going away. It was time to step inside their circle.

CHAPTER 12

Teeing Off from the Back Nine

Our family was growing. In 1990, our daughter Nicole was born, and within a few years our family of five was nearly bursting at the seams. We needed a bigger house.

I had my eye on the Emerywood neighborhood in the northwest part of town, near the golf course and country club. Emerywood consists of bigger and older homes, all stately, with massive yards and long drives. It is where the wealthiest residents of High Point live, the business owners, the doctors, the gentry. There was only one problem: it was difficult to buy into the neighborhood at the time because property was passed from generation to generation. Naturally, I wasn't about to let them shut the door on me. I fully intended to raise my family there.

I also fully intended to buy the nicest house possible. The closer a house in the neighborhood was to the golf course, the pricier it was. So I drove around looking for the biggest house I could find for sale, one as close to the golf course as possible. I saw one large brick house of about eight thousand square feet on a quiet cul-de-sac with a beautiful yard well over an acre, backing up to the country club's golf course. The tennis courts and the swimming pool were within walking distance—I would join the country club, and then I could play tennis anytime, and our family could swim whenever we wanted, without having to deal with maintaining a pool. It was just what I wanted.

When I looked up the property records, I learned that it had six bedrooms and five bathrooms, the perfect size for our family. Even better, I was happily surprised to discover that it had been built in 1970 by the banker who had started High Point Bank and Trust.

As I always did, I included in my daily prayers—which were now twice daily—my appeal to God to bless me and my family with our dream home.

Then, by chance, I learned that a colleague of mine who was a native North Carolinian was also interested in the house. That seemed to be the final nail in the coffin—he bought it out from under me, so I resigned myself to the fact that the home wouldn't be mine. My prayers would not be answered this time.

Shortly after, as I was making my rounds at the hospital one day, I was talking to another colleague who knew of my disappointment, when we saw the man who bought the house standing at the nurse's station.

"Go talk to him," my colleague urged me. "Go on, talk to him."

"What do you want me to talk to him about?" I asked. "Why would I tell him I want to buy his house when he just bought it? That would be admitting my defeat."

"Not necessarily," he said. "At least give it a shot."

He was right. I had to at least try. So I walked over to the nurse's station and struck up a conversation. I told him I'd learned we were both in the market for the same house, a topic we laughed about as we shared our appreciation for its many fine features.

He listened to me with great empathy, and as we talked, I made my proposal.

"Would you consider selling this house to me?"

He was clearly surprised, but I sensed he saw an opportunity to profit by a quick turnaround of the property.

"I might," he said, and our negotiations commenced. And before long, my family and I were walking through the front door of that house, one of the first families of color in the neighborhood.

As my practice expanded, I was able to hire excellent managers and bookkeepers, who kept the business running, and physicians, who covered the clinical care, thus freeing up my own time. As a result, I became actively involved in my children's lives and education. We required each of them to take two sports, reasoning that doing so would not only establish healthy habits, but it would teach them to be both competitive and team players, while pushing themselves as hard as they could. Elise played soccer and tennis, and Anthony and Nicole played soccer and basketball. We were soccer parents before there were soccer parents.

We attended every single game they played, and I scheduled my clinical hours around their sports schedules. If the game was at 3:00 p.m. in a distant town, I'd take off early and drive them to the game. We never missed a game, and I was still able to care for all my patients.

But sports came second to school, and they had to do well in school. They all went to private school, one of the nicest and best in the area, with excellent faculty, small class sizes, and the best resources available to them. I insisted they always be two years ahead of their class. If they were entering first grade, they had to be doing third-grade work the summer before. I helped them study, helped them with their homework, and played games like Brain Quest to test their knowledge and keep it fun.

While I considered raising them bilingually, I didn't want to create too much complexity in their lives, given how active everyone already was. Moreover, they were mixed race, but I didn't want hybrid children, with one foot in India and another in America. I wanted them to be the best Americans they could be. And they were. They were excellent students, very bright, well behaved, as well as very kind and thoughtful.

Meanwhile, from the time we'd moved to High Point, I told myself that we would join the country club. Not only was it a marker of status that was important to me, because it meant that I belonged, but the country club also provided an important network of business and community leaders and others who could make or break a career. Given my experience with the medical community, I knew not to try to join right away. The timing had to be right.

Now, with my practice established, the time had come. I was going to join the most prestigious club in town, even if it was a club that wouldn't have me.

As far as I knew, no person of color had ever been admitted to the High Point Country Club since its opening in 1923. Although several had applied, they'd all been denied. I intended to change that. But I had to approach the application for membership in a manner that would not be rejected.

The High Point Country Club had two branches, the downtown Emerywood campus by our home and the Willow Creek campus a few miles away, with a more country setting. I wanted to join both. I had a good friend at the time who was an influential White businessman. We'd met when he was my patient, but we got along quite well and shared a mutual interest in business. While I was new—though already prosperous—he was a well-established pillar of the community and quite rich. As such, he held considerable sway among the elite in High Point.

One day he came to see me, and I broached the topic of joining the country club. "I'm going to do it," I said, my confidence strong.

"Let's sit down," he said. His tone made it clear that no matter how successful I'd become, I was perhaps more confident than I ought to have been. Joining the club would not be easy.

Over a couple of drinks, we discussed the matter.

"I think you're going to create a lot of problems when you do that," he said. I was instantly on guard—was my good friend telling me not to cross the line? But before I could say anything in my defense, he added, "Don't do anything. Let me take care of it. But just sit still. Don't do anything."

I have never been good at *not* doing something, as my entire life had been the outcome of taking action, but alas, I recognized another back door when one was presented.

"Okay," I said. "If you think you can make it happen, I'll hold off." We changed the topic and enjoyed our drinks, while in the back of my mind I was gnawing away at the thought that no matter how successful I had become, no matter how many lives I'd saved, no matter how many friends I'd made in the community, I was still going through back doors. I was still seen first for the color of my skin and judged for my accent. Yet I knew I had to persevere. I had to go through yet another back door, because it was the only way to finally reach the front door. And I knew, as well as I knew the human body, that the human spirit could not be defeated as long as I never lost sight of my destiny. And my destiny was to climb so high that I could open doors for others.

So I agreed to hold off and let my friend take care of it.

I didn't have to wait long, because the very next day he showed up with an application to the country club. After helping me with a few questions here and there, he left it for me to fill out. At first the questions were standard—my name, address, age, education, profession, marital status—but then came the loaded questions. What are my hobbies? If I'd said bowling, it would have been scrapped. Fortunately, I could confidently say I played tennis. List my banking references. Okay, done. Then came the big one—how many generations of my family had lived in North Carolina? I knew what that meant. And finally, what was my reason for joining?

I spent the next two evenings answering the questions as honestly and judiciously as I could, and on the third day, I signed it and returned it to my friend. Then, instead of submitting the application to the admissions committee directly, he spent the next couple of weeks visiting the homes of each member of the committee. There, he would not mention that he had seen anyone else, or that he planned to. He appealed to each one's individual sense of honor, speaking highly of me and all that I had to contribute to the community. And each time, he came away with their signed commitment to admit me.

By the time the admissions committee met for their quarterly meeting and my friend presented my application, it could not be denied because every member had signed their commitment to admit me. Still, I would not be admitted until I'd passed the in-person interview. I met with them for afternoon tea, and that was when they peppered me with questions about my genealogy. Who were my grandparents? What kind of family had I come from? They didn't want to hear about what a loving and good family I had come from. They wanted to know about my aristocratic heritage. And that was something I couldn't deliver.

Instead, after some talk about my grandfather's stature in our community, I shifted from the past to the future and spoke about the legacy I intended to leave for our community—the medical center I'd launched, expanding my medical practice to add more state-of-the-art buildings, making Bethany Medical Center a welcoming place for everyone.

After hours of interviews and days of waiting, my family and I were admitted to the country club, and other people of color soon followed—through the front door.

PART V

THROUGH THE POWER
OF FORGIVENESS

"The ultimate source of happiness is not money and power, but warm-heartedness."

Dalai Lama

❧ CHAPTER 13 ❧

Not to Be Denied

As we settled into Emerywood in the nineties and raised our small children, I was managing our growing real estate portfolio, and I'd even opened a modest construction company. My medical business was thriving, thanks in great part to the four pillars I had established—we would treat anyone who walked through our doors, we would expand our hours to include early morning and evening hours, we would stay open seven days a week, and no appointment was necessary. Even without an appointment, we would see anyone within thirty minutes once they walked through our doors.

Those four simple concepts made it impossible for others to compete without doing the same—and my competitors in medicine did not want to do the same. They limited their patients to those who were insured, and most kept business hours. That meant that I was busy caring for those the others would not care for.

But there was still the problem that had followed me throughout my life—being a minority. In India, I was a minority as a Christian. In England and America, I was a minority as an Indian. Once we'd moved to the South, that minority status became all the more important to how I and my family were viewed in the community. I had no interest in engaging in personal or courtroom battles and making the lives of others difficult. I merely wanted to be treated with respect—and have my family treated with respect as well. I was utterly heartbroken at the way my children and I were shunned and disparaged, but I knew that there was only one right and true response. I had to forgive them.

Since I had been a small child, my mother and grandfather had instilled in me the power of forgiveness and taught me that forgiving those who wound us is a central tenet of Christianity. But forgiving such hateful actions is not easy. Still, I knew that the only way to gain the respect of those who scorned us was to forgive them their sins. I wasn't going to leave town, and I wasn't going to fight them. I was going to forgive them, and I knew that if I did so, one day they'd come around. So I prayed with all my might to forgive them their lack of understanding.

When they demonstrated more resistance, I prayed more. Then, slowly but steadily, like a miracle, the more I focused my prayers on forgiving them, the less angry I felt and the more compassion I felt. More importantly, as I forgave them, the power of Christ reached out and touched their souls and their resentment slowly diminished, and with time, my family and I were gaining acceptance in the community that had for so long shunned us.

The result of that acceptance began to touch all areas of my life. My profits were soaring, and I was becoming an important player in High Point's business and health care sectors. Because of that success, doors were finally cracking open. True, there were many who still resented or distrusted me—resented me for my success or distrusted me for my Indian origins. But many were coming around and recognizing that I had a talent for business and making money—and they wanted to hitch their wagon to mine. I was fine with their doing so because I recognized that forming alliances in the business community would benefit everyone, including those we served in the High Point area.

It was while talking with four of these associates in the business community that I found myself lamenting the limited banking options in the Piedmont Triad area.

Having been discriminated against by the leading bank in the area myself, I knew that there must be many people in the area who longed for an alternative. Could I apply my philosophy of access to medical care to the banking industry? Could we make banking more accessible to those who weren't being served by the existing bankers in the area?

Clearly this was not something I could do on my own. Nor could any of my upscale colleagues. But together we realized we could launch a more inclusive bank. Each of us had economic resources, but more importantly, each of us had social resources as well. And so it was that in 1990, as I battled entry into the country club, we began fundraising to launch the Bank of North Carolina.

We started the fundraising program with a goal of raising $11,000,000. While that may have been quite a big goal, especially in the nineties, during the time of so many savings and loan bank failures, we knew we could do it. And sure enough, it didn't take long before we had commitments from several local investors who recognized the potential of a rival bank in the High Point area. Our efforts were so successful, in fact, that we soon caught the attention of the High Point Bank and Trust—the very people who would not give me the loan for my business. Just as they'd tried to block my success in medicine by not giving me a loan, once again they set out to block our success in banking. Their motive this time was understandable, of course. We were going to go into direct competition with them.

A hearing was called before the Banking Commission, where the High Point Bank and Trust argued that there was no need for another community bank in High Point. Given their long reach in the community, it was no surprise when the Banking Commission agreed with them and denied our request to open a bank in High Point.

Again, rather than accept defeat, we decided to find a back door. That back door was in the next town over, Thomasville, another furniture town. While the economic base of the town was built on the quality furniture they produced, there was no community bank in the city, so we applied to open one there and had no problem getting our application accepted. Thus, with the collective assets of ourselves and our investors, in 1991 we opened the Bank of North Carolina, not in any impressive high-rise, but in a double-wide trailer in Thomasville. I was put on the board of directors and appointed as chairman of the loan committee and became the largest individual shareholder. I was clearly in the inner circle of the Triad's business community at last.

In our early days, as we began approving loans from that double-wide trailer, we built our first bank building, using my construction company and drawing on my experience building my medical practice—as well as the lessons I'd gleaned all those decades before when I oversaw the construction of my parents' home. Though the scale was much grander, the basics I'd learned in turning a vision into a reality remained as true for the bank building as it had been for that humble home. Quality materials, a beautiful design, and close oversight of the expenses were essential.

Once our bank had opened, our business took off. We had a lot of local support, which helped establish trust in the community. We hired people to run the bank on a day-to-day basis, as we all had other professions, so we knew we were in good hands. We also advertised, and soon we had a lot of people depositing money with us, and we grew quickly. Once we were established, we moved our headquarters to High Point, because although we were blocked from starting in High Point, once a bank is established, it can move anywhere it wants. So like it or not, the High Point Bank and Trust finally had some competition—and nothing delighted me more than knowing the bank that had turned me away now had to compete with me for its own business!

From there we became a statewide bank, and soon we were expanding into South Carolina and Virginia. By the end of the decade, we had branches in three states and about sixty different cities. It was an amazing feat, one that put me on a crash course in finance. I took remote courses from the Wharton School of Business and others to understand more about the banking industry, as well as read a mountain of books and papers on the topic, and attended all the meetings, conferences, and association meetings I could find that addressed anything related to banking. It wasn't long before I knew as much about finance as I did about medicine.

For the first five years we held our loan committee meetings in my medical office. That saved me having to make an extra trip, and by that point, every hour saved was an hour maximized.

My decision-making in matters related to people had always served me well. I was blessed to have the right people come into my life whenever I needed them. Mr. Joseph had given me housing when I first moved to London. Sir Gray had given me prestigious work in London and entry to London's social scene, which introduced me to key players in my career at an early stage. The banker I met who had invited me to attend his course in financial planning had set me on the path to wealth. Dr. Chiles had made it possible for me to start my practice in High Point, and Don Bulla, the physician assistant I'd hired early on, remains with me to this day, after thirty-two years. Don takes on a great deal of my workload, helping me to recruit and train new doctors and run the business.

In addition to raising our children, Janice and I continued to work in real estate and manage our rental properties, and we increased our commercial property holdings. Our life, in other words, was a maelstrom of activity, but it was an exciting activity as we took on more challenges and expanded our investments and interests beyond High Point.

As our professional lives and investments grew and we settled into our lives raising our children in High Point, my daughter Shirin had been raised in England under the care of her grandmother, who was growing old. We visited as often as we could, and she began visiting us in the United States, and while our bond was as close as possible given the distance between us, it was hard having her so far away. It was becoming clear that Shirin needed to be with her brother and sisters in High Point, so when she was able to make her own decision, she came to live with us.

She immediately fit right in, and she and her brother and two sisters got along beautifully. Having been well educated in England and well raised by her grandmother, Shirin was as bright and polite as her siblings and did well in the private all-girls school where we sent her. In short, our home life was as thriving as our professional lives—and every bit as demanding.

With our family and my medical business keeping us busy but happy, the banking business began to grow beyond our expectations. We had become a regional bank, so we changed our name to reflect that expansion. The Bank of North Carolina then became BNC Bancorp. We grew the bank to $9 billion in assets, with offices in numerous cities and towns in North Carolina, South Carolina, and Virginia.

Coming out of the financial crisis of 2008, BNC Bancorp was in a great financial position. We opened many new offices and bought several other banks. It was then, to my pleasure, that we were able to buy High Point Bank and Trust, the bank that had twenty-five years ago denied my first loan in High Point. We promptly changed its name to BNC Bancorp.

We also merged with Tennessee-based Pinnacle Financial Partners and became a four-state bank. We had taken a risk in opening the bank, and that risk had paid off. The banking business proved so successful, however, that it was no longer possible to continue my role and still manage my medical practice and all my other obligations. It was time for me to step down from the bank's board. I was ready to expand into new ventures—ventures that would take me to the White House—and back to India, where I had the most important work of my life to carry out.

CHAPTER 14

Called upon to Serve

When Bill Clinton and Al Gore brought their bus tour to North Carolina in 1992, I was eager to get involved. After all, when I was a child, my grandfather's political activity and influence in Kerala had infused in me a deep sense of civic commitment and the belief that we could make the world a better place through our actions. That was the spirit I embraced as I got involved in fundraising for the Clinton campaign, never expecting that by doing so, I would find my way into the White House itself.

The invitation for the two-hundred-plus Christmas party came by way of a phone call, followed by six weeks of waiting for my security clearance. They walked me through every step, until one day they told me I had been cleared and sent me a badge that would get me in. We were told where we would be staying—at a hotel next to the White House, where all the other guests were staying. When the time came for the event, we walked over to the White House, passing through metal detector after metal detector before we were escorted into the East Room Ballroom for the festivities.

I was in awe that first evening at the White House. I was amazed at how my life had taken me that far—and I sure had no idea at the time that it would be the first of many invitations to the U.S. Capitol, from three different presidents and two different political parties, cementing my status as a VIP in my adopted and beloved country. From then on, I kept up my interest in politics as a centrist, supporting different presidents.

By the time I returned to High Point after that first White House event, I knew that it was time to use my money and success to give back to those who were not as fortunate as I had been. By this point, I was wealthier than I'd ever imagined.

Every business I had established had been profitable, and all my prayers had been answered. I had a wonderful family. I was a successful doctor. I'd established a thriving medical clinic, a lucrative real estate company, and a bank that was rapidly expanding. But I knew that God wanted more from me. God had not blessed me with such wealth and success just for my own benefit. It was time to return to India and invest my wealth where it really mattered—in the children who, like me, had been born into poverty and longed for a future they deserved.

I had returned to India many times since coming to America, and we took the family on vacations throughout the world. They were growing up to appreciate not just their rightful place in America, their native home, but their rightful place as citizens of the world. Yet for all our travels, it was to North Carolina, and to High Point, that my soul always returned, not the land of my birth.

It had been decades since I'd left India, and I had no desire to live there again. Yet a question increasingly gnawed at me. Why had I been born in India? What was my purpose there? Just as there was a reason for my success, I knew that there was a reason for my birth in India, even though I had always felt uncomfortable in that environment, as if I didn't really belong there. The way I have always operated—my way of thinking, my very nature—was not very Indian at all. I was far more Western, far more cosmopolitan in my outlook and behavior. Yet I was born into that mystical land where poverty and hunger went hand in hand with a culture of celebration. Of all the places on earth, why had God ignited my life in India?

I needed to do something. I couldn't just walk away from India any more than I could return to India to live. Clearly God had arranged for me to first open my eyes in Kerala. Now that I was in North Carolina, he wanted me to open my eyes once again. It was up to me to give back a portion of blessings to the land of my birth.

I could have written a check to the United Way or some other charity and felt good about it. I could have made a donation to a local university, as so many people do. But I felt I needed to do something deeper, something more meaningful and long-lasting, instead of just sending a series of checks.

I also felt compelled to do something for my faith. As a minority Christian in India, I felt a calling to share my blessings with other Christians there. These two thoughts—doing something meaningful and long-lasting, while also sharing my blessings with other Christians in Kerala, coalesced in my mind for weeks, until I reached the point where I knew I had to return to India and search for an answer. I knew that if I sought the answer, God would direct me.

The plane set down at Trivandrum Airport. I passed through customs and greeted my brother, George, and my sister, Gladis, who were awaiting me. We drove to George's home in Kerala and caught up on what each of us had been doing. George was married with children and well established in his career in education administration; Gladis was happily married to the doctor we'd found for her and had just returned to India after living in Africa for several years. As always, it was a treasure visiting my family and former home, but this time I wasn't there for socializing. I had work to do.

I met with the priest at St. Anthony's Shrine and explained to him my desire to help the people of Kerala. His warm smile told me I had come to the right man.

"God has sent you to us, Lenny," he told me as he poured us some steaming-hot tea from a silver teapot. He sat back in his chair and continued as we sipped the comforting beverage. "There are so many children here in Kerala, children just like you once were—bright, curious, playful. But unlike you, they have no future. Some have parents who cannot care for them; others have lost their parents to sickness or accident. We care for them at a nearby orphanage, but we do not have the resources to provide much for them. We cannot afford to give them the education their minds deserve. Indeed, it is a struggle just to clothe and feed them. If you could help these orphan children, God would bless you even more than he already has. Can I take you there?"

I met his smile with my own. I could think of no better way to give back to God than to care for his orphaned children. Finishing my tea, I said to the priest, "I would be so happy to meet these children and learn more."

We arranged for a visit to the orphanage the following day, and I arrived promptly, so eager I was to meet not just these unfortunate children, but to meet my own future as well.

My driver took us up a windy road through the lush and gorgeous hills of Kerala, until we came to a modest blue and yellow building adorned with a statue of Mother Mary. Over the door was a sign that read the Jayamatha Boys Home. A group of boys was playing football in the courtyard—what we call soccer in America. Their laughter was so refreshingly musical, but it quickly silenced when they saw the shiny chauffeured car pull up and the priest and I emerged.

Instantly, I was surrounded by the curious faces of the boys, who, rather than beg for alms like in the city, remained polite and welcoming. Yet I could not help noticing that they were indeed poor, their clothing ragged and ill fitting. I knew instantly that any help I offered them would be well spent.

We went inside, where I met with the administrator, a Jesuit priest, and I told him of my grandfather's school and what good memories I had of his efforts to help and educate the youth of Kerala. After some discussion over another pot of tea, I was shown around the building and introduced to the nuns and monks who taught the children, as well as the children themselves, who mostly giggled or hid their heads in shyness. I was so touched and, at the same time, so transformed to know that I could put my wealth to such a noble cause.

"I'll tell you what," I told them after a long conversation about their needs (which were great) and their assets (which were not as great). "I can give you the financial support you need and help you to expand your services."

Their joy was uncontained. "Dr. Peters, that would be a most generous gift. Thank you and God bless you," the priest said, as others in the meeting joined in with their gratitude.

I was thrilled to put my wealth to such a worthy cause, but at the same time, I wanted to be sure that my money would be well spent. So I added, "In return, I would request a few things."

"We would be delighted to hear you out," the priest said. I could tell that he was both cautious and excited. I continued.

"I want a role in directing it," I said. "I don't want to interfere with the good work you're doing, but I'd like to put someone in to oversee the finances and make sure it's well organized."

I watched as he shifted uncomfortably in his seat, no doubt concerned about losing control over his school. But that wasn't my intent at all. He could continue to run the school, but with the money I was prepared to invest, I wanted some fiscal oversight. I needed to know the money would not be spent frivolously.

"I want you to hire more employees and expand your reach throughout Kerala. And I want whatever we do to be lasting. So I will commit to funding your program throughout my lifetime and thirty years after my death."

The smiles that radiated from each priest's and monk's face made it clear—we had a deal.

With the expansion of the Jayamatha School for Boys, my life was changed. I was able to turn a struggling orphanage into a vibrant community that served the needs of those who most needed it. I was also giving back to God, as we introduced Christianity to these unfortunate children. We do not convert them, however. We don't even require that they be Christian. We take in children from all faiths. But we raise them in a Christian environment, so that when they reach the age of eighteen, they can make the choice to convert on their own or not.

The purpose of the homes is not only to give the children a home and education but to also train them in a trade so that when they leave the home, they will be able to find work. But they are not forced out when they turned eighteen. If they need to stay a few more years, they can. There is no urgency. We want them to be safe, and we want them to be prepared for the world. And we realize that some children are slower than others in gaining their independence, so they need more time.

Best of all, since I have become involved, one out of ten of those children has gone on to become a Christian missionary—which is the ultimate reward in my eyes, as I have helped spread the word of Jesus Christ through these wonderful homes for orphaned children.

But as we got started expanding the school in those early days, there was only one problem. Sending money to India was not easy. The complex financial system for getting money in or out had long been a source of frustration over the years, as I regularly sent my family money. And while I did want a role in overseeing how my money was spent, I did not want to be there managing it or have to deal with opening accounts in my name just to ensure the orphanage received the money. I wanted to establish a foundation that would provide the framework for funding the orphanage. Through a foundation, I would be able to easily send money to India while still retaining control over it. But again, there was a problem. I was busy enough as it was. I didn't have time to run a foundation. I needed someone else to manage it. And I had just the person in mind.

Gladis and her husband had spent much of their married life raising their children in Africa, where he had a medical practice, and traveling around the world. Now that her children were older, she was ready to settle down and had essentially retired early while her husband had scaled back his practice to part time. They were well off—not only did they own Bethany, the home I had built for my parents and we had bequeathed to her and her husband as part of her dowry—but they also had a home in the city, a couple of cars, and a couple of servants. They were well off by Indian standards but not wealthy by American standards. I needed a bright, capable person I could trust to run the foundation, and Gladis was just that person.

So one day I said to her, "I want you to work for me."

In response, she laughed. "Lenny," she said, in a tone to imply I'd asked her to clean my house, "I don't want to work! And I don't need the money! I'm enjoying life and keeping busy. Why would I want to go back to work?"

Now it was my turn to laugh. "I didn't say I would pay you, Gladis! You just have to work for me. Everyone needs a purpose. You have to justify your existence. Just think of what it would mean to help these children!"

Perhaps she was offended at my directness in implying she had to justify her existence, but it was true. Gladis was a wonderful woman, with so much to give. It seemed wasteful to have her gifts and not put them to bettering the world, which I knew in her heart she wanted to do. We had remained close throughout our lives, so I knew her love for me would help her to make the right decision.

"Okay, okay," she said. "What do you want me to do, Lenny?"

"I want you to be the president of the Lenny Peters Foundation in India and run it for me," I answered. I wasn't just asking for her help. I was offering her an opportunity I knew she'd jump at, despite her initial reluctance to go back to work.

I didn't have to wait for her answer. The pride on her face made her answer clear. "Okay, I'll do it," she said, and with those words, our work began.

After I had my attorneys and accountants set up the foundation in the United States, Gladis took charge, and we expanded to India. She recruited employees and volunteers, and though we didn't pay much, we had no problem finding people with graduate degrees to join us, some even quitting high-paying jobs in order to join our cause. The

Lenny Peters Foundation was established to be purpose-driven, which means everyone who comes to work for us is motivated by that purpose, rather than the financial rewards.

Once we had a core group of skilled people, we began talking to as many priests, monks, and nuns as we could, and they eagerly joined us, which enabled us to expand our mission throughout different parishes, finding children who were in need of housing and education, as well as adults in need of medical care or financial aid. Of course, as in any new effort, we made mistakes. We initially distributed medications, food, and clothing, but we discovered that the clothes didn't always fit, and the food often couldn't be eaten because it required cooking and they didn't have the means to cook. Too much was going to waste. So we finally figured out that if we just gave them an envelope with cash, they could get what they needed and the waste problem was solved. People who don't have enough to eat or who are ill do not blow their money. They meet their needs first. And that was our goal.

As word of the foundation spread, so did the need. We were soon branching out throughout the region, and our volunteers would travel to remote villages, and with the help of local parishes and priests, they would find people who were dying or in need of health care. We wanted them to know that there were people who cared about them. For those people, we don't just dispense money. Our volunteers spend time with them in their homes, keep them company, help them as needed, and sometimes just listen.

We also put together a program of prayer, where a priest or nun would visit someone who was seriously ill and pray for them. That program proved quite effective, because the simple act of prayer expresses unconditional love and gives hope to those most in need of it.

Next, and most importantly, we established an orphanage for girls. Mother Teresa's orphanage was only about two miles away, which is why we didn't initially establish one. In India, it would be unheard of to house the boys and girls together, and since they knew how to monitor and care for the girls, it seemed best that they do so while we cared for the boys. But when a building became available, we renovated it into a nice modern building. Once we had enough experience, we were more confident in caring for the girls, and it was clear that for all the efforts of Mother Teresa's orphanage for girls, there was a need for even more care. There were just too many young girls in need of homes and education. Thus, we established the Lenny Peters Home for Girls.

In giving the home my name, my intent was not to boast but to brand the charity, as well as ensure that if I solicited donations for the school, people would know that it wasn't some abstract faraway enterprise. If I asked for donations and my name was on it, people knew they could trust their donation would be well invested. And my children and grandchildren would also be more inclined to support the school after my death, if it bore our foundation's name.

I had seen both successes and failures in that regard with my friends whose children showed no interest in continuing the good works of their parents. But when a family's name is attached to a cause, the children are more likely to take an interest in it. So with the branding of our girls' orphanage as the Lenny Peters Home for Girls, I was confident that no matter in which directions my children might go after my death, they would have a personal interest in keeping the home going. I couldn't have asked for a more noble legacy.

Although I had always been generous with my wealth, with the formation of my foundation and establishing the home for the girls, it wasn't only Gladis who had a newfound purpose in life—I did as well. The Christian tradition has always made generosity of spirit and wealth a foundation and helping the poor a commandment, and the more that I followed those precepts, the more I understood the wisdom behind them and felt the touch of the Lord. That touch became an embrace as time passed, bringing me even closer to the good Lord.

One day I had the good fortune of meeting the archbishop of the diocese in Kerala. He arrived with an entourage of attendants and, after shaking my hand, invited me into the dining room for afternoon tea. As we sat down, he reached across and held my hand. A moment later, he said, "I feel something." Before I could ask what, he asked his entourage to please leave us alone for a couple of hours and requested that all his appointments be canceled. "I'm just feeling something so different," he again told me once they had left.

Over the next two hours, we talked about Christianity with a depth and spirit I had rarely experienced. I was in the company of a truly holy man, and he clearly recognized in me something of the Divine Spirit as well. After that first meeting, we met again several times, and he taught me a great deal about the history of Christianity in India. Through our many meetings, we grew close, and I knew that I could always count on the archbishop for any assistance he could provide, should I need it.

In kind, I gave to his convents and hired his sister as the chief nun at the Home for Girls. By that time, we were caring for close to one hundred and fifty boys and thirty girls, while providing care for twenty to thirty others each day. Whenever I have needed any assistance, the archbishop has been true to his word and helped me with whatever influence or help he could provide.

It was through the archbishop that I gained the trust of everyone throughout the region, and that trust proved to be invaluable one day when we were approached by a group of physicians and nurses who were caring for terminally ill patients in the last years of their lives. They knew of our work and my close connection to the archbishop, and they trusted that we could help them. Their organization was floundering, and they knew they needed to restructure their work or they would have to abandon their efforts.

I heard them out and saw that they were indeed dedicated but overwhelmed by the task before them.

"All right," I assured them. "If you're prepared to restructure everything, I will fund it." And that is how the Lenny Peters Home for Palliative Care came to be.

My life's purpose had blossomed beyond anything I had imagined, and as it did, my relationship with God grew ever deeper.

CHAPTER 15

Success, Excess, and the Power of Self-forgiveness

The nineties was a decade of prosperity and success for me, one that continued into the new millennium, as my businesses flourished, I opened a new clinic in High Point, and I continued to invest in, and raise funds for, the foundation. But such success comes at a price, and I was paying that price.

The children had all grown up and gone off to college, and our once hectic family life began to settle down. I had spent so much time working, however, that once the children were older, it was clear that Janice and I had grown apart. We still shared a bond and a great respect for each other, but our lives had diverged. My focus had been on work, and my marriage suffered for it. We also had different visions for our future. Finally, in 2007 we agreed to divorce, so one Friday evening I moved out of the house in Emerywood and into a two-bedroom corporate apartment in Greensboro.

At first it was disheartening to find myself alone in such a small, generic apartment, but I was determined to make the best of it. Though I was never much of a drinker and never went downtown to bars—I'd never even been to a club in High Point before—I was suddenly single and ready to enjoy a night out on the town. So the next day, I ordered a black limo to pick me up in the early evening.

I dressed up and was ready to go when the driver came to the door. He was a young Black man, and he introduced himself as Idris.

"Nice to meet you, Idris," I said. "Take me to the best nightclub in town," I said. "What do you suggest?"

"Well, the best one in town is called Heaven," Idris replied. "On South Elm."

"Then take me to Heaven," I directed. I couldn't have asked for a more auspicious beginning to the evening.

As we drove to what he assured me was a popular and elite club, we chatted amiably. After some conversation, he asked, "Do you mind if I ask you, sir, how you became so successful? I haven't met many minorities who have attained your status here. Where did you come from?"

In reply, I told him a bit about my life story until we pulled up in front of the club. "Thank you, Idris," I said as I bade him goodbye. "Have a nice evening."

"Sir," he responded, returning my tip, "I'm so fascinated by your story that I'm going to stay right here. I want to take you back home."

"No, you go home," I encouraged him. "I'll be here quite late, I'm sure."

"No," he insisted, "I'm going to call in and clock out. But I'll be waiting here when you get out."

It was apparent that there was no talking him out of it, so after pressing the tip into his hand once again and wishing him well, I went inside. My driver had been right. The club was a spectacular one—three floors, each one packed with well-dressed partygoers.

I asked the hostess, "Who owns this place?"

"Joey is the owner," she said.

"Can I talk to him?" I asked her.

A look of concern crossed her face, no doubt worried I was going to complain about something, but she stepped away, and shortly after, a relatively young, clean-cut, and well-built man came down the stairs and introduced himself to me as Joey. I told him who I was and explained that, like him, I was a local businessman and entrepreneur and was quite impressed with the nightclub he'd established. He invited me to join him for a drink, and I learned that he'd had a rather unconventional entry into the nightclub business, coming from humble beginnings and eventually acquiring four clubs and restaurants in the Greensboro area. He'd been so successful transforming the seedy downtown into a popular nightspot that his nickname was the "mayor of downtown Greensboro." The "mayor" clearly had a knack for business and making his customers feel at ease.

Joey gave me a tour around the club, and it was even more impressive than my initial impressions. The first floor was an upscale Caribbean-type tropical bar that served colorful fruity rum cocktails in tasteful glassware. No tiki bar, this one, but with a real island vibe, complete with reggae music. On the second floor was a restaurant, again upscale, and on the third floor was a rooftop nightclub with a spectacular martini bar. I spent some time there and had a great experience.

When I finally called it a night, it was nearing midnight. When I stepped out the door, there was Idris, waiting just as he'd said he would be. He drove me home, still asking me questions, and as we pulled into the drive, he said, "Sir, I want to quit my job and work for you. You don't have to tell me what you'll pay. You just pay me whatever you think is right."

And with that, he quit his job with the limousine company, and Idris has been my trusted personal driver ever since.

After all those years with a large and active family, those early days of our divorce were emotionally brutal, though I did my best to avoid those emotions. My sadness was made all the more painful with the death of my beloved mother in 2008. Shortly after the time my parents stayed with us briefly when we first moved to North Carolina, my father died and my mother returned to live with us, and she became as much a part of the family as my wife and children. Now, however, she was gone. She chose to be buried in High Point, near my home.

The laughter and easygoing conversation of my home life were replaced with the silence of living alone, and the large, luxurious home was replaced with the sterile white walls and temporary furniture of my corporate apartment. I felt as if I'd fallen backward in some respects, living in an apartment much like the one I'd had in Pittsburgh. Back then, of course, such living was fine, wonderful even, as I was young and just starting out and compared my standard of living to what I had grown up with. Now I compared it to all that I'd achieved and how I'd been living for more than two decades, and the contrast was profound. I spiraled downward into a spiritual darkness and sought solace in the most efficient way possible—returning to the club.

I returned to Heaven the next week and the week after that. It took only a few visits for everyone there to know my name and greet me as if I'd been a regular for years. After only two weeks, I said to Joey, "I want to buy this place."

Joey smiled and said, "Sorry, Lenny, but I'm not selling it."

I smiled back and replied, "Joey, you don't know it, but in two weeks, you're selling this place, and I'm buying it."

We shared a laugh, but just as I'd predicted, within two weeks I had persuaded two of my partners in one of my business ventures to join me in buying the building and all three businesses for around $2 million.

Joey Medaloni was happy, and so was I. Heaven was mine.

It never would have occurred to me that I'd end up in the restaurant business, but there I was, owner of the hottest nightspot and restaurant in town. We decided to keep everything pretty much the way it was, but we changed the restaurant's focus to Italian food, and the decor to more of a South Beach meets Mulberry Street decor. I had the entire top floor remodeled, with private booths curtained in ethereal white gauze, and the beautiful waitresses wore wings—we called them angels. I built a special VIP area with cabanas and added a big two-story DJ booth, with dueling DJs. A big screen showed music videos for the songs the DJs selected, as the crowd—there was always a crowd—danced away.

I didn't have to do much myself. I hired managers to run the businesses, and after working all day at the clinic and finishing up my administrative work, I'd return home, take a nap until about 8:00 p.m., shower, put on my best clothes, and Idris would arrive in the limo I'd rented. By 9:00 or 9:30, we'd pull up in front of the club, and the place would already be packed, with lines of people around the block waiting to get in on the weekends.

I'd be escorted to the front by one of the two bodyguards I'd hired, walking through the doors like the most important man in the city. Everyone wanted to join me in my cabana, but not everybody could. The cost just for entry was $500, yet every evening there would be ten to twenty people paying the entry fee just for the status of being seen in my cabana. Beyond the cabana, there would be up to four hundred people on the rooftop alone. The money rolled right in.

I felt as though the dark days were lifting, but the truth was, the dark side was pulling me into a spiritual vortex that threatened to devour me. But at the time, I didn't see it that way. I had money and no one to answer to. The kids were far away, in other towns and states. I had a limo, a driver, and even bodyguards—one in the front and one in the back. If there was any trouble, they nipped it in the bud. I didn't even have to worry about imbibing too much, because Idris would drive me home and see me inside each night. I was living the dream, in my own Mar-a-Lago.

I was also hitting rock bottom spiritually yet telling myself I was having the time of my life. In truth, I longed for the stability and comfort I'd once had. The dueling desires for an unrestrained life of nightly decadence and the calming comfort of family and home battled within me. Although I never doubted for a moment that ultimately I'd return to the stable life I felt I was losing, I couldn't help but delight in the nightlife I hadn't enjoyed since my younger days. Rather than sell my stake in the business, however, I bought out my partners and became the sole owner.

I kept up this life for more than two years, during which time my divorce with Janice became final. She stayed on as president of our real estate business, and we agreed to split everything evenly. We also agreed that I'd buy her out of her share of the house. She was happy with the money, and I was happy to be back home.

All the while I kept up my crazy lifestyle. I never took a woman home from the nightclub or did anything improper, because I wanted to maintain my professional image. But it was still a lifestyle that lured me into a hedonistic outlook that was far from my spiritual roots. I loved the lavish, celebratory nightlife; the prideful feeling that came from being surrounded by so many people vying for my attention; and the constant flow of money. That money, however, wasn't always reaching me or my partners. Although we were raking in up to fifty grand a night on a busy weekend, and a respectable gross on week-nights, it wasn't long before I realized that some of my managers and workers were skimming off the top. The money wasn't counted until around 3:00 a.m., after we'd closed and long after I'd gone home, so it was easy for them to help themselves to a pile of bills each night. Once I'd realized what was going on, however, I couldn't fire them because we needed them. I did not have the time, much less the experience, to run a nightclub and restaurant. Even to replace the managers would not only mean a setback in having to train a new crew, but there was also nothing to prevent those new employees from doing the same. So I accepted that the skimming was another cost of doing business, and besides, I wasn't in it for the money. I was in it for the sheer pleasure it brought me.

It was that sheer pleasure that was doing me in. My kids first noticed it, and my friends and business associates as well, and they let me know they were concerned about what they viewed as my midlife crisis. My friends would say, "You've never acted like this before."

Initially I ignored them, but night after night of such a life soon catches up to you. Being back in my home helped to ground me. Ever so slowly, the life I was living no longer brought me joy. Ever so slowly, I realized I'd given in to the temptations of pride and hedonism. God pulled me away from the darkness and returned me to my true nature—as his child and witness, one who had a greater purpose than dancing away the nights. After nearly three years of playing Gatsby, I found myself in spiritual darkness. I had hit rock bottom but hadn't even realized that was where I was heading because the ride down had been so fun. But I wasn't having fun anymore. I was living the life of a superficial attention seeker while no longer experiencing life, just celebrating an escape from it. Realizing the joy those nights once brought me had long passed, I finally accepted the fact that my Heaven had become my Hell. So just as quickly as I'd bought it, I sold the restaurant and nightclub, but I kept the buildings, so the rent—which couldn't be skimmed—kept rolling in.

❧ CHAPTER 16 ❧

The Power of Prayer

It was during these years, as well, that I returned both to the White House and to my spiritual roots. My success in business had enabled me to both attend and host fundraising events for candidates of both parties, which in turn expanded my social network and brought me immense pride as I actively contributed to American democracy.

The days of being shunned by my neighbors and colleagues were increasingly behind me. While the subtle slights from the few would never go away, almost everyone looked up to me as a business leader who had led the revitalization of the High Point health care system.

My foundation was also thriving, and the continued letters and cards I received from grateful children whose futures had been secured by safe housing and good education had brought me incomparable gratitude. They also brought me closer to Christian leaders in India, whose guidance I truly needed in the wake of veering into the darkness of my nightclub days.

After I'd returned to my home, as thrilled as I was to be back, it just hadn't felt the same. It was just me alone in all those rooms that had once been alive with voices and activity. Of course, I could have sold the house, but I had battled to get into that neighborhood—my home in Emerywood was a part of my soul. I wasn't leaving. But I did need a change. I decided to remake the interior, transform it from "ours" to mine.

I set about remodeling it. With the help of some designers, I updated everything, added some modern lighting and furnishings, and by the time it was done, I felt as if I'd bought a new home and never left home. It was wonderful. But the most important change was I added a prayer center, where I could pray and worship as I returned to my spiritual journey.

I became close with a priest from India and invited him to stay at my home so that we could discuss our shared spiritual interests and pray together. I was building worship centers in India as my way to give thanks to God for all my blessings and do my part to bring Christianity into the lives of other Indians. We organized spiritual retreats of two days to a week, where people came from throughout India and ate, prayed, and stayed together in pursuit of their own spiritual healing.

These retreats were so successful that I organized one in High Point and invited a number of my most influential friends to attend. Among them was an Indian cardiologist from Detroit who flew in for a weekend retreat. We were speaking before the meeting, standing quite close together, when I noticed he was holding his right arm close to his body, as if it was injured.

"Have you injured your arm?" I asked him.

"My rotator cuff is shot," he said. "That's why I'm here. I can't even lift it. I can't do anything with it. It's essentially paralyzed. I had to quit my job seven years ago because I had no functional movement. It's just never healed. So I came here to pray about it."

I touched his arm. "Let's go inside and pray," I suggested.

We stepped inside the prayer room, and I joined him in praying for his shoulder to heal and enable him to return to work, so that he could return to saving lives.

The next morning, a Saturday, we gathered for communal prayer and the priest began chanting and chanting, as the energy in the room grew greater with every chant.

"Hallelujah! Hallelujah! Hallelujah!" everybody shouted in reply to the priest's melodious chants. I was caught up in the elation myself as I cried out, "Hallelujah!" in adoration to God for his divine presence and all the blessings he had bestowed upon us. As I did so, I caught sight of the Indian cardiologist and saw that he, too, was crying out "Hallelujah"—his hands raised high in the air in praise to God.

I was shocked. This man had left his profession because he couldn't move his shoulder, and after we prayed together just one time, his paralysis was gone. I did not know if it was psychological—his belief in the Holy Spirit so great that it overcame the pain and restored his shoulder—or if the Holy Spirit had indeed entered him. But I knew that with the power of prayer, one man had been healed so that he could return to his calling and heal others through his gifts as a skilled cardiologist.

My devotion to God and return to my spiritual roots showered me with a spirit and enthusiasm so much greater than my wild nightclub adventure. I had been excited running the nightclub, thrived on the attention it brought me each night, but my spirit had never felt that excitement. This was an entirely different experience—now I thrived on the blossoming of my spirit, and the powerful feeling of my union with God grew more intoxicating every day. My connection to God became so much closer, my purpose so much clearer. I had been given the gift of healing, of transforming people's lives, and now that gift was being opened to the world. My faith and devotion were enabling me to touch people's lives in ways I never had before. It was a remarkable awakening.

Having been so awakened, I made my office at Bethany Medical Center a space for prayer and spiritual reflection. No one was expected to pray, but being in the Bible Belt, almost everyone who worked for me was a Christian. It wasn't unusual for a few people to follow me into my office each morning and join in a common prayer. There was enough space for each person to quietly say their special intentions, and then one of us would lead the prayer. I even had Bible cards on my desk, like playing cards, but with Scripture on one side and a prayer on the other. Each morning, as we prepared for our prayer, I would randomly pick a card and give it to someone in the group to read aloud. We even read from the Bible every day. It wasn't long before our medical team was bonded not only through our work but through our devotion to God, and that bond helped our powers of healing in remarkable ways.

At the same time, our staff are trained physicians, nurses, and technicians, and the health care we provide is the best that medical science has to offer. But the best is not always good enough. I wanted our clinic to offer not just the best medical care, but to be a part of cutting-edge research in cardiovascular, endocrine, gastrointestinal care, and others—such as infectious disease, pain studies, and disorders of the central nervous system. So in 2006, I founded Peters Medical Research. PMR works with pharmaceuticals to provide Phase II, III, and IV clinical trials—the clinical trials with hundreds of participants once a medication or device is found to be safe for people. With about one thousand people walking through our doors each day, we had the perfect opportunity to recruit participants. Opening our services to provide our patients the chance to participate in these drug trials has enabled many to take lifesaving drugs that would otherwise not be available to them. And it has contributed to the scientific knowledge that is so necessary for medicine to advance.

Putting my trusted associate, Don Bulla, in charge, I was able to maintain my focus on clinical care and management, while knowing my scientific interest in research and invention would continue.

I have always been respected for my medical skills, but prayer and devotion seemed to enhance those skills, and others began to notice as well. From the very beginning, when I first began studying medicine, I felt as though I had a different touch. I could actually feel when I was healing someone, as if I was somehow imparting my spirit through my touch. Of course, the gift of healing is well known in India, but in the United States, many remain skeptical that spiritual power can exist alongside science. Yet as one who is well trained in the scientific method, one who is firmly convinced in the power of science, I can say with equal certainty that certain spiritual gifts are every bit as powerful as even science—and sometimes more so.

Over the course of my career, it was not uncommon for people to come see me for a second opinion after receiving a dire diagnosis. I could put them through the same tests their previous physician went through, the same ultrasound or the same endoscopy, for example; have them take the same medicines and follow the same course of treatment; and have entirely different results. Just placing my right hand on their left shoulder and assuring them, "We're going to heal this. We're going to get you better," was often all it took for my patients to feel hopeful, and so many times, that's exactly what happened—their illness disappeared. Perhaps it was their optimism once I'd given them hope that helped heal them when nothing had worked before. But as I've looked them in the eye and assured so many of my patients that they'd get better, I have felt the energy transfer from me to them, as if the energy is almost flooding them through my hand, the conduit. It is for that reason that I believe it was the power of prayer and my close connection to God that has helped so many of my patients to heal and is one of the reasons I have had such a flourishing practice.

One experience that stands out was receiving the call that a patient was gravely ill. She and her husband were both close friends and patients, and she had been hospitalized for severe necrotic pancreatitis. Her pancreas was effectively dying—which meant that she was dying. Her blood pressure had dropped dangerously low, and I was summoned for surgery. I opened up a bile duct—a small tube connecting the liver to the pancreas—which I hoped might drain some of the bile salts and ease her pain. The operation was a success, but she still had a difficult time ahead of her.

Around 2:00 a.m., I was called back to the hospital because she was collapsing. I knew the chances of her survival were slim, so I wasted no time. I sat by her bed and pumped the IV fluid as quickly as possible, adding more fluid, pumping it in, adding more, pumping it in, hoping to stabilize her blood pressure. I kept it up for close to an hour, but

I was determined she would survive. She woke up around daybreak, looked at me with confusion, and said, "Lenny, what are you doing here? You should be home sleeping."

I don't think I'd ever been so happy to see a patient wake from such a close brush with death. She later explained that she had passed through the tunnel—she had indeed been dying. But as she realized the determined efforts we were making to save her, she came back—and to this day remains a loyal friend.

Several of my patients have spoken to me about seeing the tunnel. One woman we brought back from near death who was suffering from lung disease told me, "I went through this tunnel and I looked, and there was Dr. Peters, sitting with God. And Dr. Peters and God both told me to go back, so I went back through the tunnel, and just like that, I'm alive. It's weird."

I don't know how many thousands of lives I've saved over the years, but time and time again, after all the objective testing possible, just in a sense, I have discovered the cause of a patient's suffering. It might be colon cancer just about to invade and metastasize, and we've found it, cut it out, and cured them completely. Or it might be a lesion on a lung or a heart disorder—something that the objective tests have missed, but an overpowering sense that we should look again or look elsewhere has enabled me to save a life that otherwise would have been lost.

Given these many experiences saving the lives of my patients in High Point, it's not uncommon for me to be driving through town and spot someone playing tennis, for example, and think, *That man is playing tennis because of me*, or spot a familiar child on the way to school and think, *That child is walking into school because of me*. The gift that God gave me to heal has been the finest gift he's bestowed on me, far greater than all the success, the wealth, and the opportunities. And for that gift, I've seen to it that my practice gives daily thanks.

Among the steps I took to express that gratitude was to have all my white jackets embroidered with the words "I treat, God heals." At first my staff was shocked, but my associate, Don Bulla, had the same words stitched onto his jacket, and a few others did as well. We understand that we can only treat our patients, but the healing comes from God. These words that initially shocked some have now become a sort of motto at our clinic.

In my many years as a physician, I have come to understand that healing is not something I can do alone. No doctor can. Healing is an act of God, and when I place my hand on a patient and assure them, "We will heal this; you will get better," I am telling them that I will work with God to heal them. When I invited a group of priests from India to start their missionary work here, they visited my clinic, and the power of God was palpable.

They told me that they felt unusual energy everywhere they went in the clinic, as if God was walking alongside them, as if he were there, in every room, seated beside every bed. They returned to India and told others of it, even went on tours on four or five continents, telling people that there was a doctor in America who healed through God. That is what I do.

Now every building in Bethany Clinic has a photo of me, and beneath each photo, it reads It's HIS work I do.

Some people might say of me, "But he's a scientist! How can he believe such things?"

And to that I say, "If you really want to see oxygen before you breathe it, go for it."

God has been by my side for many decades now. He has brought me unbelievable riches both in wealth and in family. But the gift of healing he gave to me is a gift that will forever extend God's love far beyond my humble life. By giving me the gift of healing, God has given others the gift of life.

And for that I bow down in prayer and gratitude.

CHAPTER 17

A Legacy of Love

My children grown, my businesses prosperous, and my medical practice, research center, and foundation continuing to touch the lives of thousands from North Carolina to India, it became time to reflect on all that I had built up in the decades since I first left home, walking across those rice fields with my father and two small bags. In those years I had amassed a fortune, lived a life of luxury and splendor, and most importantly, returned in kind the many blessings God had bestowed on me by improving and saving the lives of friends, strangers, patients, children, elders, and everyone in between.

I couldn't have imagined a better life, and even my darkest days were blessed. And while advanced in years, I felt as much youthful vitality as I had in my forties. Yet the tides of time were moving fast, and I knew that I had to do something to prepare my children for the responsibilities ahead of them after I passed. I had not built up such a business empire only to have it all dissolve once I was gone. I wanted the foundation to continue, my clinics to live on, and all my holdings and investments to continue to provide for my family and others for generations.

Shirin had graduated from New York Medical College, gone into private practice with me in High Point, and married a fellow doctor, J.R., who is an intelligent and kind-hearted young man. He is an assistant professor at New York University and conducts research in visual rehabilitation. Shirin very much wanted to return to New York, so to get her started, I helped her open a Bethany Medical Clinic in Manhattan. In short order, she and her husband loved New York and had an established life there, with no desire to return to North Carolina. Her desire to stay in New York distressed me, as I wanted her to take a role in the businesses in North Carolina, but I also knew that she is passionate about her life in Manhattan, and I had to accept that. Since then, I have remained very supportive of her efforts, and she has grown Bethany Medical Clinics to several locations in Manhattan.

Anthony has also excelled, graduating from the University of Pennsylvania and Wharton School of Finance with a dual degree in finance and biomedical engineering. Having started out in consulting in New York, he realized his true love was medicine, so he began applying to medical school, while Nicole studied international studies at Duke University. Though she had started out with a keen mind for business and the ambition to match it, as time went on, she realized she wants a more creative life.

And Elise went into business, graduating with a bachelor's degree and later an MBA from the Wharton School of Finance, marrying and having a baby girl. Elise's husband, Matt, is a gifted young man with an MBA also from Wharton. He started his own company in insurance technology, of which he is the founder and CEO. Elise moved to New York, as well, and worked for American Express and Capital One, where her skills in finance, market data, and capital management proved exceptional, and she showed great interest in learning from me as well.

My children have met and exceeded all my expectations for them, and every opportunity I had to be with them was cherished. But there often comes a time when the children are grown that a parent has to talk business, and that time had come for me. I called everyone together for a series of family discussions and presented them with my plan.

My own death does not frighten me, as my devotion to God has instilled in me a sense of peace and the certainty of an eternal hereafter. But the death of my businesses is unthinkable. It is important to me that whenever I shall pass, it will be knowing that I've left my businesses in good hands. Each of my children has the potential to gain the experience and expertise to ensure the many investments and holdings we have will live on, yet none necessarily has the desire to do so, as they have established their own lives. And so it was that when the children were all living in New York, I began having meetings with them on Sunday afternoons at a second home I'd established in Manhattan.

Those Sunday afternoons were devoted to business discussions, where I would tell them about everything I'd done in terms of our investments. At the time, the children were still rather young in their adulthood. They didn't understand real estate; they didn't understand finance. They had no idea how vast my investments were, nor how many assets I'd accumulated. So those weekly meetings were an opportunity to educate them, prepare them for their future as active participants in the business, and, eventually, as inheritors of the estate.

Finally, one day, it was time to tell them my plan. "Here's the deal," I told them. "I'm proud of each of you, but with the blessings you've enjoyed come responsibilities. I'm not going to be one of those parents who works like a dog while their kids are having a great time living off that work."

I saw a few eyes roll and some shifting in their seats, but at least I had their attention. I then said, "I want a written proposal from each of you about what you're going to do to help me build the family business. It has to be in writing and make clear what you want and what you're willing to do to make it happen. And then I'll consider it and decide what I'm willing to give. If we can make a deal, we'll make a deal. Otherwise, I love all of you equally, but I'm going to make my own decision about what I do with the family business and with my life."

There was some grumbling, but I wasn't having any part of it. "That's the way it is," I said, making it clear that I wasn't budging. I could see that they were clearly struggling with the prospect of return-ing to High Point and working in the family business. Shirin loved New York and didn't want to leave. Anthony had his heart set on medical school, so he was unable to join me, and Nicole was so young at the time that she was just finding her place in the world. Only Elise was in a position to take my offer seriously. And only Elise did so.

It was after several such meetings that Elise came to me with a writ-ten proposal. She proposed returning to High Point and learning the family business and managing with me. With her MBA from Wharton and the experience she'd been getting in finance while working in New York, I was confident she was just the one to do it, but still, I knew she was young and would need some training. So I accepted her proposal, and she returned to High Point with her family.

Elise and I attended several courses in business and finance and joined an international group of advisers to family businesses. We talked with accountants and attorneys, and by the time we were done, she had learned even more than she'd learned at Wharton.

When I was confident that she was ready to take on the respon-sibility of managing so many different enterprises and such a large investment portfolio, we met with attorneys and I had a legal docu-ment drawn up that gave her a large share of the company in ten years. Then, when I pass away, she would control the businesses. The other children would be taken care of as well, but because she was devoting her time and career to the business, she would receive the majority.

Elise wasn't the only one to move back and work with me, how-ever. Her husband, Matt, is to be commended for supporting the family by first splitting time between New York and North Carolina and ulti-mately moving to High Point full time. It was a great sacrifice on his part, and I congratulate Matt for being part of a great decision to move to High Point, and I am all the more delighted because I can now spend time with their three children, Adeline, Isabel, and Edward.

Shirin remained in New York with her husband and their two children, Cosimo and Soma. Anthony graduated from medical school at UNC-Chapel Hill and completed his residency at the University of Virginia, where, like me, he was chief resident. After that he started his fellowship training in cardiology at Duke University. He married a delightful young woman, Ashley, who is caring and compassionate, with a master's degree in counseling. Ashley took a job in Durham as a professional counselor, and they have two children, Charlotte and James. Anthony is now as busy as he is happy to be working so close to home and in such an esteemed position. And Nicole, too, returned to High Point and joined Bethany Medical as an information systems analyst, a position she's been brilliant at.

But only Elise has shown any real interest in growing the business, so she and I worked side by side, growing all the more close and all the more serious about safeguarding the fortune—and reputation—that I have achieved in my lifetime.

And during all these changes, another president was inaugurated, and again I was invited to the White House, this time with an invitation to join the president and vice president themselves for a more intimate gathering. This time I had no need to shop for a new tuxedo, as the designer came to me. This time the president would so admire my jacket that he'd want one made just like it. I had come such a long way from my early years walking barefoot to school. Now I was admired by the most powerful man in the world, dined with dignitaries, and discussed the future of the world with the wealthiest, most influential men and women in America. I controlled a vast real estate portfolio, owned several medical clinics serving a thousand patients a day, was founding director and chairman of the loan committee of a bank that had grown to four states and remained a major shareholder. More recently, I became co-chairman of a bank, Carolina State Bank in Greensboro. I directed a foundation that helped North Carolinians in crisis, housed and educated orphans in India, and helped spread the word of God.

How far I had come since moving to North Carolina, when business leaders shunned me, denied me loans and housing, urged their patients to avoid me. The clinics I established were named "Family

Business of the Year," by the *Triad Business Journal*, and I, one of the "Most Admired CEOs." The Chamber of Commerce named Bethany Medical Center "Business of the Year," while the *Triad Business Journal* honored me as one of the "Top Ten to Watch" among "Power Players" and recognized Bethany Medical Center as one of the Triad's "Fastest-Growing Companies." I was no longer viewed as a dark-skinned immigrant who didn't know his place and didn't belong. I had found my place, found my sense of belonging.

Yet I longed to see my grandfather's face once again, to see in his face the pride I knew he would feel for me. He never could have imagined all that I'd achieve, but it was his belief in me, his conviction that I was born for something great, that had started me on my journey of success.

And it was my belief in God and Christ and my conviction that they'd blessed me for a greatness I could only vaguely fathom as a child that gave me the courage to take that journey—a journey whose destination I have yet to imagine. In some ways, I am only getting started.

CHAPTER 18

A New Beginning

It might be hard to imagine now, but 2020 started with a great beginning. Our businesses were doing well. Elise, now fully engaged, began running things as president of the company. Bethany Medical was again recognized as one of the *Triad Business Journal*'s Fast 50 companies, the top 50 fastest-growing companies in the Triad region. Everything we had been working toward was coming together.

For me, personally, I finally had some free time. I began traveling often to my home in Miami Beach, enjoying the sunshine and the many facilities associated with the resort. I had a tremendous time, all the while working remotely with Elise, building the family businesses. I had even found a new personal trainer, Gui, a bodybuilder from the West African country of Niger, who has won several national championships. We bonded not only as trainer and client, but spiritually. He and his wife own a boutique gym, where I would go early every morning at six o'clock to work out with him, sometimes starting our workout with a prayer. He and I are still in great health. After a full checkup recently at an anti-aging institute, I was told I was getting younger rather than getting older. I was seventeen years younger than my biological age. I felt good; things were going in the right direction.

January and February flew by. Bethany Medical had moved its headquarters downtown to a newly renovated office building that we bought, and our forty-five-member team, including many of our senior managers, had already moved in. Our banking and development interests were also taking off.

Yet, as we now know, there was great disruption on the horizon. On the other side of the world, a virus had begun to spread, first throughout Asia and then to parts of Europe. By March it was clear that this novel coronavirus we had been hearing about for months was working its way from Wuhan, China, around the globe and would soon be upon us, too.

I was at my home in Miami Beach on a Saturday in mid-March when the vice president of my organization called me and said the governor was going to close the schools in North Carolina because of what was by then being called COVID-19.

"Okay," I said, "I'm on my way back. I'll be there tomorrow." I knew that this looming pandemic was going to require a fast and effective response from our clinic, and we needed to be at the forefront of protecting and treating our patients.

We had an emergency meeting of our senior management on Sunday night. We started to put strategies into place to fully protect our employees and continue to see our patients. We realized we were at the frontline in the war against this virus. We immediately started our own COVID-19 testing lab. We decided to fight this monster head-on rather than fighting from behind. While other health care providers around us were forced to suspend certain services and rededicate hospital space to treating COVID-19 patients, we adapted from within. We never closed our offices. We were already seeing nearly nine hundred patients per day come through our doors prior to the pandemic. Once the pandemic took hold, we began to see more than one thousand patients through our doors each day—about an 11 percent increase.

At Bethany Medical, we kept our clinics open seven days a week. In June, in the middle of the pandemic, we opened our new location in the nearby town of Kernersville. That new clinic took off and flourished. During July and August, toward the tail end of the first wave of the pandemic, at a time when most businesses were closing down or laying off their employees, we hired 142 new employees across our companies, including doctors, nurse practitioners, and members of our senior management team. We would not lay off anyone, but we would be safe, so of course we took precautions—wearing masks, social distancing, washing hands, and not congregating in large groups. As a result of these precautions, we did very well through the pandemic. Sadly, however, the impact of the pandemic would affect millions of Americans who fell sick or the hundreds of thousands who died, as well as so many more around the world who have suffered from this deadly virus.

In the midst of crises, though, it is my belief that we must look for the silver linings to be had. And in that regard, it is a credit to our employees and our senior management that Bethany Medical had its best year in thirty-four years of operation amid the pandemic. A lot of that success has been due to our hard work and the momentum we established prior to 2020, and it just so happened that a lot of what was already in motion came to fruition at that time. Still, even with all the progress and the juxtaposition of it all transpiring throughout the world's greatest health care challenge in more than a century, I wanted to do more.

I marvel at how my life is now, compared to the days so long ago when I was driving around London in a TR7, living it up and exploring the nightlife across the water in France or even owning my own nightclub in downtown Greensboro so many years later. While I thought at the time that I was living my best life, I now feel far more joy and I take so much more pleasure today in my family, as well as in the security I—and now with the help of my children Elise and Nicole—am working to provide for our future generations.

That security extends to our community as well. As I write this, we have twelve development projects in and around downtown in the works. These projects are, with the spirit of forgiveness in mind, all working toward a goal of making the city of High Point, particularly its downtown, a more attractive area for residents as well as industry and business. Therefore, I have decided to participate as much as possible in the revitalization of downtown.

We will see how the pandemic will shape the future of corporate offices and how people commute to work and perform their jobs, but I still envision downtown High Point as a place where young professionals and empty nesters who have recently retired, or will soon do so, will flock to live. I understand the pandemic has sent a lot of people back into the mode of looking for rural living spaces and maybe has even led some renters to buy whereas before they had considered themselves not yet ready. But prior to the pandemic, the youth and the retirees across the United States were moving more toward downtown living, seeking to be near the staples that support a healthy, balanced lifestyle, including all the amenities, entertainment, retail, and groceries that an urban environment can provide. I am still convinced, even more so now, that once the pandemic is behind us, this will be more true than before. People will seek what they have been denied, and there will be many who have had time to prepare their finances for such a move. What's more, just as I believed the South to be a good place to invest in my own real estate holdings, as the East and West Coasts become increasingly prohibitive for young adults and retirees to find affordable housing, the South becomes all the more attractive for both its affordability and its beauty.

We have seen the same trend in our commercial interests. By the time it's all done, our portfolio will have invested about $60 million into the downtown area, some in commercial office space and other holdings and some in residential and mixed-use, commercial and retail space.

My faith, which has guided me to make all these decisions in my career and to develop the relationships with people who have helped me along the way, is even stronger today. The saying goes "Luck is where opportunity meets preparation." In addition to the orphanages we run in India, our foundation now has one in Africa and another that will open soon in South Africa to be run by my niece, Susan.

Again I marvel at how far I have come and how far I have yet to go. The businesses are healthy, as are my children and grandchildren. Our family continues to grow, as does our presence in the community in High Point and our charitable interests around the world.

I have had so many kind souls come into my life, so many blessings that I cannot account for my success other than to say that, along with hard work and a competitive desire to always do my very best, I have relied on my faith and the power of forgiveness to guide me in my decisions and in my relationships. I have not always made the right decisions. I have failed and felt shame and embarrassment as all humans do. But I have never given up, never lost faith, and never been too proud or felt too put upon to forgive.

I am invigorated today by the promise of tomorrow, and through it all I believe the best is yet to come. I am far from finished. I have said before that I feel as though I am not nearing the end of my journey, but rather, I am just getting started, and I am not alone in my journey. My family, from the departed to my living family—my children and grandchildren, my siblings and their kids—we are all together just getting started!

EPILOGUE

My Personal Message to You

It seems today that the world is at odds. Everyone is angry with each other or fighting with one another because each of us has been hurt, treated badly, or harmed in some way. And much of this has to do with our personal histories, how our parents or our ancestors were treated either in this country or in our native countries, which, like myself, so many have taken the leap of faith to leave behind for greater opportunities abroad.

In my travels across four continents, learning and practicing medicine, I have discovered this to be true. There is no place in the world, nor are there any people, immune to the fact that past hardships existed, inflicted on us by our neighboring nations, our own countrymen, or sometimes our own families. This fact, to varying degrees, of course, is universal.

My message is this: there is more to gain than there is to lose through the power of forgiveness. Had I fled North Carolina when I was met with so much resistance, I have no doubt I'd be a bitter man today. But I had confidence in myself and in my inherent worth, so instead, I faced those who saw only the color of my skin or heard only the accent in my voice. I also had confidence in the inherent worth of those who feared me, because I knew that their prejudice was not based on their experience with people who differed from them but on their lack of experience. They may have lived in the same community as people of color, yet they had little experience working, living, and worshipping side by side with them. As they came to work, live, and worship with me, they came to respect me. In turn, I learned to forgive them their fears and inexperience, and as I did so, my own heart opened to them.

It is crucial that we recognize—and this idea is not particular to any one race or ethnicity or country, but to mankind—that we cannot turn back the clock. We must focus on today and instill in our children the confidence and faith to be more open and welcoming to those who differ from them.

We can all have the same opportunities today, though I recognize that for some of us, those opportunities can only be accessed through a back door. Access through traditional means may at some point be denied to us, but one who is motivated will always discover an alternative way in. I built my entire legacy by doing so.

Is somebody denying you something that you desire? If so, it is up to you to find a way around the obstacles they've placed in your way. If not, consider drawing on the power of forgiveness to release you from your anger and frustration. I believe your good fortune will be returned to you manyfold if you focus on the power of forgiveness and have faith in yourself. Your faith does not have to be strictly a religious faith, but a belief in yourself and the people around you, in your fellow man, and in the universe. All of that will return to you in the form of a large magnitude of energy.

People often talk about good energy and bad energy. Let me tell you how you create good energy in your life. You wake up each morning, positive about the day ahead, knowing that the universe is on your side. You are not thinking about what happened one hundred years ago, one hundred days ago, or even one hundred hours ago. Focus on what's ahead of you, not behind you.

We are not consumed with the obstructions in our path as we rise to brush our teeth, throw together a quick breakfast, and get the kids off to school. If we can prevent these obstacles from creeping into our thoughts as we head out the door to meet the demands of our day, we can surpass them.

I am not preaching a philosophy I have not lived. This has been my experience. I have been adamant about this tenet even as I raised my own children. I made it a point to take my children on the physical journey to see firsthand my poor beginnings. I made each of them walk the same walk, carrying a bag, that I had made with my father when he sent me off to premed at fourteen. I wanted them to know firsthand the feelings I had on that momentous day.

I brought them to my family home in India, where I lived as a young boy with my mother, my brother, George, and my sister, Gladis. I laughed when they asked me, "Where is the house?" and I replied, "You're looking at it."

It wasn't much of a house to speak of. But I wanted them to see that. And I wanted them to see St. Anthony's Shrine. I did all of this so they could see and experience with their own senses their roots and the climb I had made to shield them from the kind of poverty I and my family knew at that time.

Yet I never sat them down to speak about the hundred years of British domination of India, the atrocities committed, the pilfering of our lands, resources, and labor. I never instilled in them a sense that we needed to feel vengeful about the history of colonialism in my native land.

In doing so, my children have grown up with a sense of normalcy, a sense that they can accomplish anything they set their minds to do, and they were not inhibited in any way by the past. I took it even one step further. If my children were going to be raised in America, to be Americans, they were going to be the best Americans they could be.

Instead of raising them in one language in the home and teaching them strictly about India in the home and then sending them out into the English-speaking landscape around them and confusing the children before they even became teenagers, I elected to raise them in a more balanced fashion. You can't ask children to have one foot in one boat and the other foot in another boat and expect them to move forward. The boats will inevitably stray in two different directions.

To decide, as an immigrant, to be here in America, you must decide to be the best person you can be. To come here, I had to decide, what is the purpose in going to America? That doesn't mean I gave up on my culture or feel no pride in my heritage. I am proud of my Indian compatriots, our contribution to today's world, and all the success some contemporary Indians have achieved. The CEO of Microsoft, the CEO of Google, the CEO of Pepsi-Cola, and even our incoming vice president are all Indians or of Indian heritage. We are doctors, lawyers, business leaders, and movie stars. So I am proud of our culture. My point is we do not need to dwell on our weaknesses. That is not how any of us who have succeeded have accomplished our goals or achieved our positions in life or in America.

Were we to continue to focus on our weaknesses, we would only serve to raise a weak group of people in our future generations. Everyone asks me how I raised four very different children who are each so amazingly talented. My response is always the same. I did not raise them. God raised them. I was raising God's children.

In my journey to discover who the British people were who had conquered us and how they seemed to have so easily dominated my native country where they were so outnumbered, I discovered that British people are not inherently bad people. They are good people, and for all their wrongdoing, the truth is that the British did contribute greatly to the modernization of India. They built the railway system uniting the North and the South, the East with the West. If not for this amazing infrastructure, India might still today be a series of small, opposing countries, without direction. They also taught us English, gifting to us the universal language, which has played a key role in our rise as participants and leaders in the global economy.

And while I was in the U.K., sure, I did face discrimination, but I also met some truly great people. One, a well-educated and in fact knighted distant member of the royal family who befriended me and helped me at no great benefit to himself. Had I been focused on the wrongs done to my country by the British aristocracy, I would never have been able to enjoy the gracious gifts Sir Gray bestowed on me professionally and socially.

The lessons I have been fortunate to learn in my lifetime, on four separate continents and in fields ranging from medicine to real estate to banking and now construction and development, have all come to me accompanied by the kind and generous souls sent to me without my doing, and through the power of forgiveness instilled in me so many years ago as I knelt beside my mother in prayer beneath St. Anthony's Shrine.

It is my hope that what you have read here, or will read here, serves as motivation to you, regardless of your own background. There is nothing a person cannot do if his or her intentions are right and the hard work is done, because all of us are surrounded by those who have the means, the desire, and the opportunity to help. No one makes their way in this world alone. Nor does one succeed for long without mastering the power of forgiveness.

"Never give up; there is always a back door."
Lenny Peters, M.D.

ABOUT THE
LENNY PETERS FOUNDATION

Established in 2006, the Lenny Peters Foundation is proud to be a helping hand in North Carolina and around the world. The foundation provides charitable grants or donations to needy individuals and families in the Piedmont Triad as well as to many other charity organizations in the USA. A firm believer in philanthropy, Dr. Peters recognizes his humble origins.

Through the Lenny Peters Foundation, he has formed and is currently financing the following centers: the Jayamatha Boys Home, India; Lenny Peters Home for Girls, India; Lenny Peters Home for Palliative Care Center for the Terminally Ill, India; Lenny Peters Prayer Center, India; Lenny Peters Home for Children, Johannesburg, South Africa; Lenny Peters Divine Mercy Home, India; Lenny Peters Home for Child Protection, India; and Lenny Peters Home for Family Welfare, India.

One hundred percent of the proceeds from the sale of this book will go to support orphaned children and cancer patients through the Lenny Peters Foundation.

Dr. Lenny Peters credits his deep-rooted Christian faith, his mother's devotion, and his grandfather's example of giving back to his community as the tenets that have kept him grounded throughout his successful career. Not yet finished, Peters has turned over all businesses to his capable daughter, Elise Peters Carey, and is now focusing his time and energy on his family, community, and charitable interests. For more information about the foundation, or to contribute, please visit lennypetersfoundation.org.